T0259514

Burnout in Nursing: Causes, Management, and Future Directions

Editors

GEORGE A. ZANGARO
DOROTHY DULKO
DEBRA SULLIVAN

NURSING CLINICS OF NORTH AMERICA

www.nursing.theclinics.com

Consulting Editor
BENJAMIN SMALLHEER

March 2022 • Volume 57 • Number 1

ELSEVIER

1600 John F. Kennedy Boulevard • Suite 1800 • Philadelphia, Pennsylvania, 19103-2899

http://www.theclinics.com

NURSING CLINICS OF NORTH AMERICA Volume 57, Number 1
March 2022 ISSN 0029-6465, ISBN-13: 978-0-323-91972-2

Editor: Kerry Holland
Developmental Editor: Axell Ivan Jade M. Purificacion

Nursing Clinics of North America (ISSN 0029-6465) is published quarterly by Elsevier Inc., 360 Park Avenue South, New York, NY 10010-1710. Months of issue are March, June, September, and December. Periodicals postage paid at New York, NY and additional mailing offices. Subscription price per year is, $163.00 (US individuals), $689.00 (US institutions), $275.00 (international individuals), $710.00 (international institutions), $231.00 (Canadian individuals), $710.00 (Canadian institutions), $100.00 (US and Canadian students), and $135.00 (international students). To receive student/resident rate, orders must be accompanied by name of affiliated institution, date of term, and the signature of program/residency coordinator on institution letterhead. Orders will be billed at individual rate until proof of status is received. Foreign air speed delivery is included in all *Clinics* subscription prices. All prices are subject to change without notice. **POSTMASTER:** Send address changes to *Nursing Clinics*, Elsevier Health Sciences Division, Subscription Customer Service, 3251 Riverport Lane, Maryland Heights, MO 63043. **Customer Service: Telephone: 1-800-654-2452** (U.S. and Canada); **1-314-447-8871 (outside U.S. and Canada). Fax: 1-314-447-8029. E-mail: journalscustomerservice-usa@ elsevier.com** (for print support) and **journalsonlinesupport-usa@elsevier.com** (for online support).

Nursing Clinics of North America is covered in *EMBASE/Excerpta Medica, MEDLINE/PubMed (Index Medicus), Social Sciences Citation Index, Current Contents, ASCA, Cumulative Index to Nursing, RNdex Top 100,* and Allied Health Literature and International Nursing Index (INI).

Contributors

CONSULTING EDITOR

BENJAMIN SMALLHEER, PhD, RN, ACNP-BC, FNP-BC, CCRN, CNE
Associate Clinical Professor, School of Nursing, Duke University, Durham, North Carolina

EDITORS

GEORGE A. ZANGARO, PhD, RN, FAAN
American Association of Colleges of Nursing, Washington, DC

DOROTHY DULKO, PhD, ARNP-BC, AOCNP, WHNP-BC
Lead Core Faculty, Graduate Program, American Association of Colleges of Nursing, Washington, DC

DEBRA SULLIVAN, PhD, MSN, RN, CNE, COI
Senior Core Faculty, College of Nursing, Walden University, Minneapolis, Minnesota

AUTHORS

MARY A. BEMKER, PhD, PsyS, CNE, RN
Quality Matters Peer Reviewer, Usiu Reiki Master and Teacher, Henderson Fellow, American Association of Social Psychiatry Fellow, College of Nursing, Graduate Program, Walden University, Minneapolis, Minnesota

BONNIE DIPIETRO, MS, RN, NEA-BC, FACHE
Director of Operations, Maryland Patient Safety Center, Elkridge, Maryland

AMBER DONNELLI, PhD, RN, CNE
Walden University, Minneapolis, Minnesota

DOROTHY DULKO, PhD, ARNP-BC, AOCNP, WHNP-BC
Lead Core Faculty, Graduate Program, American Association of Colleges of Nursing, Washington, DC

CHRISTINE FRAZER, PhD, CNS, CNE
Senior Core Faculty, College of Nursing, Walden University, Minneapolis, Minnesota

MARCOS GAYOL, EdD, MSN, MPH, RN, CNE, CPH
Dean of Nursing and Health Sciences, Aspen University, Denver, Colorado

VINCENT P. HALL, PhD, RN, CNE
MSN Program Director, Walden University, Asheville, North Carolina; Walden University, Minneapolis, Minnesota

VICKIE HUGHES, DNS, MA, RN, CENP, FAAN
The Johns Hopkins University School of Nursing, Baltimore, Maryland

VICTORIA HUGHES, DSN, MSN, RN, FAAN
Assistant Professor, The Johns Hopkins University School of Nursing, Baltimore, Maryland

JULIE JAMES, MSLIS
Walden University, Minneapolis, Minnesota

BETTY J. KOHAL, DNP, PMHCNS-BC
Walden University, College of Nursing, Minneapolis, Minnesota

TRACY LOOKINGBILL, DNP, MSN, RN
Program Director, Aspen University, School of Nursing and Health Sciences, Denver, Colorado

JEANNE MORRISON, PhD, MSN
Nurse Executive Academic Program Coordinator, Walden University, Hattiesburg, Mississippi

LYNN C. PARSONS, PhD, RN, NEA-BC
Professor and Department Chair, Department of Nursing, Morehead State University, School of Health Sciences, Morehead, Kentucky

ROBIN SQUELLATI, PhD, APRN
Core Faculty, Walden University, Minneapolis, Minnesota

DEBRA SULLIVAN, PhD, MSN, RN, CNE, COI
Senior Core Faculty, College of Nursing, Walden University, Minneapolis, Minnesota

VIRGINIA SULLIVAN, MA
Research Assistant II, General Pediatrics, Department of Pediatrics, Vanderbilt University Medical Center, Nashville, Tennessee

DEBORAH WEATHERSPOON, PhD, MSN, CRNA, CNE, COI
Senior Core Faculty Nurse, College of Nursing, Walden University, Minneapolis, Minnesota

KATHLEEN M. WHITE, PhD, RN, NEA-BC, FAAN
Professor Emerita, The Johns Hopkins University School of Nursing, Johns Hopkins University, Baltimore, Maryland

DEBRA ROSE WILSON, PhD, MSN, RN, IBCLC, AHN-BC, CHT
School of Nursing, Austin Peay State University, Kingston Springs, Tennessee; Walden University, Minneapolis, Minnesota

GEORGE A. ZANGARO, PhD, RN, FAAN
American Association of Colleges of Nursing, Washington, DC

Contents

> Nurses experience high levels of burnout, and this has become a major factor in recruitment and retention of nurses. Several factors have been associated with burnout, but it is not clear which factors are the most significant predictors. Understanding the most prevalent factors that are associated with burnout will allow for the development and implementation of interventions to ameliorate and/or reduce burnout in the nursing workforce.

> Burnout syndrome within the early career nursing population is an issue that impacts not only the individual but also impacts the workforce, the organization, and patient care. Components of burnout are associated with 3 main areas and the contributing factors to burnout can be addressed at the individual, organizational, and institutional levels. Efforts to reduce the contributing factors and improve work satisfaction within this population will have a lasting effect on early career nurses' commitment to the profession.

> Nurse burnout is a serious global problem that is associated with adverse job factors. In this article, research on burnout as measured by the Maslach Burnout Inventory is reviewed from 2000 to 2019, specifically analyzing job factors associated with nurse burnout and comparing US with international findings. Most of the reviewed articles found a significant relationship between nurse burnout and a nurse's intention to leave their job, job stress, nurse satisfaction, and workplace violence. There were very few articles reporting on research done in the United States, whereas most of them described international research. Recommendations on how to decrease the risk of nurse burnout are summarized.

Burnout is a condition resulting from chronic workplace stress that has not been effectively managed, described in 3 dimensions: (a) feelings of energy depletion or exhaustion, (b) increased mental distance from one's job, and (c) reduced professional efficacy. Burnout is a widespread problem reaching concerning levels among health care professionals, with more than 50% of physicians and one-third as many as 80% of nurses reporting symptoms. The National Academy of Medicine (NAM) action collaborative on clinician well-being and resilience has prioritized exploring ways to enhance baseline understanding of clinician well-being and promotion of multidisciplinary solutions to burnout.

Health professionals, including nurses, are vulnerable to burnout, which occurs when chronic stress is not managed. COVID-19 led to nurses working in stressful environments, and being required to work mandatory overtime. The result was an increase in burnout. Nurses exhibited physical, psychological, emotional, and behavioral signs of burnout. There are several ways that nurses can mitigate the situation and have more control over burnout. Nurses need to work together to support each other, including supporting the leader. There are several actions, such as mindfulness activities and maintaining a healthy lifestyle that can help prevent burnout.

Pandemics are not new, but our global community allows the spread of disease to occur much more rapidly than ever before. The recent COVID-19 pandemic has placed nurses on the frontlines caring for contagious and acutely ill patients. Nurse burnout is not new either; however, these demands have put a strain on nurses, and nurse burnout has been reported as being at high levels. This article looks at a history of pandemics and examines the research related to nurse burnout during previous and the current COVID-19 pandemic. The authors conclude this article with recommendations for evidence-based interventions to decrease factors associated with nurse burnout.

Burnout syndrome has been defined as a state of chronic stress characterized by high levels of emotional exhaustion and depersonalization with low levels of professional efficacy. The effects of nurse burnout include poor job satisfaction and turnover. Nurses' physical and mental well-being are both essential to sustaining a healthy nursing workforce with factors such as an empowering work environment showing positive effects on reducing burnout. Formal and informal individual and organizational approaches to supporting novice nurses' transition and experienced nurses' sustained practice fulfillment are key to addressing burnout and fostering retention.

NURSING CLINICS OF NORTH AMERICA

SERIES OF RELATED INTEREST

Critical Care Nursing Clinics of North America
https://www.ccnursing.theclinics.com/

THE CLINICS ARE AVAILABLE ONLINE!
Access your subscription at:
www.theclinics.com

Foreword

Impact of Career Burnout Across Nursing

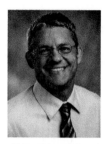

Benjamin Smallheer, PhD, RN, ACNP-BC, FNP-BC, CCRN, CNE
Consulting Editor

Discussions surrounding burnout within nursing have increased significantly. Nursing burnout has been associated with an increase in nursing turnover and financial demand on health care facilities and health systems to onboard and train new staff.[1] Burnout is found across all care settings: acute inpatient care, primary care, public and community health, nursing leadership, and nursing education. Furthermore, an individual's length of time and seniority within nursing does not provide a safeguard from burnout. Early-, mid-, and late-career nurses are reporting that their profession no longer provides the satisfaction it once did.

Many factors can lead to burnout among nursing professionals, including emotional exhaustion, depersonalization, poor social climate/social support, value incongruence, feelings of low personal accomplishment, low control over the job/decision latitude with perceived high workload, and low rewards.[2,3] The detrimental effects of nursing burnout can include reduced job performance, poor quality of care, poor patient safety, negative patient experiences, and adverse events, such as medication errors, infections, and patient falls.[2]

Finding interventions to help nurses manage burnout, create restorative environments, and improve patient safety and quality of care has been challenging; however, strategies are being explored regarding the development of resilience and support for cultural change as well as interventions specifically related to meaningful recognition, shared decision making, and increased leadership involvement and support for nurses.[4] Although much of the current level of burnout can be attributed to the increased demands on nurses created by the COVID-19 pandemic, our discipline and profession will continue to be challenged with demanding work conditions fueled by short staffing, long hours, and future diseases or hazardous situations. As a nursing community, we must work together to ensure healthy, safe, and supportive

Nurs Clin N Am 57 (2022) ix–x
https://doi.org/10.1016/j.cnur.2021.12.001
0029-6465/22/© 2021 Published by Elsevier Inc.

environments for nurses; positive outcomes for the patients and families for whom we provide care; and a sense of gratification and trust in our chosen profession.

This issue of *Nursing Clinics of North America* investigates nursing burnout and its impact throughout health care systems through a variety of lenses. This intentionally broad approach is designed to offer an expansive foundation for readers seeking a deeper understanding of the phenomenon of burnout. We have provided several articles that focus on how to reduce exhaustion and fatigue and collaborate with others who may be experiencing burnout.

Benjamin Smallheer, PhD, RN, ACNP-BC, FNP-BC, CCRN, CNE
School of Nursing
Duke University
307 Trent Drive
DUMC Box 3322
Durham, NC 27710, USA

E-mail address:
benjamin.smallheer@duke.edu

REFERENCES

1. Nursing Solutions Inc. 2021 National Healthcare Retention and RN Staffing Report. 2021. Available at: https://www.nsinursingsolutions.com/Documents/Library/NSI_National_Health_Care_Retention_Report.pdf. Accessed November 18, 2021.
2. Dall'Ora C, Ball J, Reinius M, et al. Burnout in nursing: a theoretical review. Hum Resour Health 2020;18:1–17.
3. Monsalve-Reyes CS, San Luis-Costas C, Gómez-Urquiza JL, et al. Burnout syndrome and its prevalence in primary care nursing: a systematic review and meta-analysis. BMC Fam Pract 2018;19:59.
4. Adams A, Hollingsworth A, Osman A. The implementation of a cultural change toolkit to reduce nursing burnout and mitigate nurse turnover in the emergency department. J Emerg Nurs 2019;45(4):452–6.

Preface

Understanding and Managing Nurse Burnout

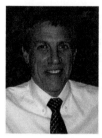
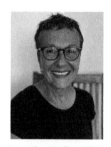
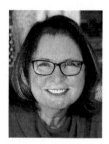

George A. Zangaro,
PhD, RN, FAAN

Dorothy Dulko, PhD,
ARNP-BC, AOCNP,
WHNP-BC

Debra Sullivan, PhD,
MSN, RN, CNE, COI

Editors

Burnout among nurses has been present for many years. During the COVID-19 pandemic, burnout was intensified by extremely stressful work environments, the emotional strain associated with witnessing increased mortality of patients, continual stress of working long hours in understaffed units, the physical strain of constantly wearing personal protective equipment, and having limited opportunities for rest and recovery between shifts. This supplement issue of *Nursing Clinics of North America* consists of 11 articles that discuss various aspects of burnout in the nursing workforce. The articles presented here reflect the diverse elements of burnout among nurses and are characterized into three general themes: (1) factors associated with burnout, (2) impact of burnout on quality of care, and (3) recognition and management of burnout.

Several factors contribute to nursing burnout. This *Nursing Clinics of North America* special issue presents factors such as heavy workload, poor work environment, low job and career satisfaction, intent to leave, and high job stress as the most relevant predictors of burnout. The findings from these articles illuminate the fact that burnout in the nursing work environment has reached unprecedented levels, having significant negative implications on the nursing workforce. Future research should aim to gain further insight and a better understanding of how these factors might be managed more effectively, including and identifying how nurses can use positive coping skills to reduce the incidence and effects of burnout.

Future research is needed to determine if burnout causes diminished quality of care or if working in a setting with lesser quality of care contributes to burnout. Understanding the nature of this relationship is critical to identifying where to allocate resources and focus interventions, improving quality of care and decreasing burnout.

Nurs Clin N Am 57 (2022) xi–xii
https://doi.org/10.1016/j.cnur.2021.11.012
0029-6465/22/© 2021 Published by Elsevier Inc.

nursing.theclinics.com

This issue also includes studies that suggest approaches to recognize burnout and provides methods for managing and reducing burnout at the individual and organizational levels. Strategies are presented for reducing early-career burnout, managing leaders who are experiencing burnout, implementing strategies to adapt and be resilient in a multidisciplinary team, reducing the impact of burnout on health, and identifying how leadership style will influence burnout. Several interventions are suggested to reduce nurse burnout, including mindfulness or meditation training to reduce personal and job stress, coping strategies, resiliency training, educational programs to increase confidence in nursing skills, and improved work-life balance. Organizational strategies include monitoring for symptoms of nurse burnout and creating policies to protect nurses from burnout. The majority of interventions identified in this review focus on small groups of individuals. Additional research on a broader level is needed to target organizational factors affecting entire hospital systems to be able to implement strategies effectively to reduce burnout across all nursing disciplines.

The articles presented here are essential for the well-being of nurse leaders and staff nurses. The early recognition of burnout and immediate interventions to ameliorate its effects are critical to the nursing workforce's health and the success of an organization. Nurses are at the forefront of the COVID-19 pandemic; it is imperative that they are aware of their physical, emotional, and psychological needs and that they are provided the needed support that enables them to adequately maintain their personal well-being and health. The strategies presented in these articles can guide government, health care organizations, and policymakers to develop guidelines that will promote the resilience of nurses during this pandemic and better prepare the nursing workforce for future pandemics. Nurses are the largest segment of all health professions, and the public consistently ranks them as the most trusted profession. Reinforcing the value of nurses, especially given the extraordinary demands currently being placed on them, and taking measures to promote well-being and professional satisfaction are urgently needed steps to maintain retention and quality of patient care.

George A. Zangaro, PhD, RN, FAAN
American Association of Colleges of Nursing
655 K St NW, Suite 750
Washington, DC 20001, USA

Dorothy Dulko, PhD, ARNP-BC, AOCNP, WHNP-BC
American Association of Colleges of Nursing
655 K Street NW, Suite 750
Washington, DC 20001, USA

Debra Sullivan, PhD, MSN, RN, CNE, COI
Walden University
100 S Washington Avenue
Minneapolis, MN 55401, USA

E-mail addresses:
gzangaro@aacnnursing.org (G.A. Zangaro)
ddulko@aacnnursing.org (D. Dulko)
debra.sullivan@mail.waldenu.edu (D. Sullivan)

Systematic Review of Burnout in US Nurses

George A. Zangaro, PhD, RN, FAAN[a],[1],*, Dorothy Dulko, PhD, ARNP-BC, AOCNP, WHNP-BC[a],[1],
Debra Sullivan, PhD, MSN, RN, CNE, COI[b],
Deborah Weatherspoon, PhD, MSN, CRNA, CNE, COI[b],
Kathleen M. White, PhD, RN, NEA-BC, FAAN[c], Vincent P. Hall, PhD, RN, CNE[b],
Robin Squellati, PhD, APRN[b], Amber Donnelli, PhD, RN, CNE[b], Julie James, MSLIS[b],
Debra Rose Wilson, PhD, MSN, RN, IBCLC, AHN-BC, CHT[b]

KEYWORDS

• Burnout • Nurse • Maslach • Systematic review

KEY POINTS

• Burnout is a global health concern with serious implications for the nursing workforce.
• Frontline workers are experiencing psychological, physical, emotional, and behavioral signs of burnout.
• The Maslach Burnout Inventory for Health Services Survey is the most widely used instrument to measure burnout in nurses.
• If burnout is suspected, the implementation of coping strategies such as mindfulness exercises, spirituality, cognitive adaptation, and resilience has all been shown to decrease levels of burnout in nurses.

INTRODUCTION

Burnout in the health professions has been a concern for several decades. During the COVID-19 pandemic burnout has emerged as a significant concern for nurses as well as health care organizations.[1] The demand for nursing services has increased significantly during this pandemic, and nurses have experienced increased levels of burnout and stress.[2,3]

Burnout is included in the 11th Revision of the International Classification of Diseases as a condition resulting from chronic workplace stress that has not been

[a] American Association of Colleges of Nursing, 655 K St NW, Suite 750, Washington, DC 20001, USA; [b] Walden University, 100 S Washington Avenue, Minneapolis, MN 55401, USA; [c] Johns Hopkins University, School of Nursing, 525 N. Wolfe Street, Baltimore, MD 21205, USA
[1] The views, analyses, and conclusions expressed in this article are those of the authors and do not necessarily reflect the official policy or positions of the American Association of Colleges of Nursing.
* Corresponding author.
E-mail address: gzangaro@aacnnursing.org

effectively managed. It is described within 3 dimensions: (1) feelings of energy depletion or exhaustion; (2) increased mental distance from one's job; and (3) reduced professional efficacy (World Health Organization [WHO] 2019).[4] Burnout has reached
concerning levels among United States health care professionals, with more than
50% of physicians and one-third of nurses reporting symptoms.[5] The WHO has
acknowledged the serious consequences of burnout resulting from persistent workplace stress, reporting burnout levels among physicians and nurses at new highs
and consistently increasing.[4] A recent study revealed that nearly 80% of registered
nurses experience burnout; 64% of advanced practice registered nurses and 56%
of clinical leaders also report feelings of burnout.[6] The effects of burnout among the
nursing staff has been shown to result in increased patient mortality ratios, increased
rates of hospital acquired infection, increased absenteeism, decreased job performance, and job dissatisfaction.[7–11]

The costs of burnout are not limited to affect the personal well-being of health care
workers. Research has shown that health care provider burnout can result in unsafe
patient care with higher levels of burnout being associated with increased medical errors and potentially compromised patient safety.[7,12] From the institutional level,
burnout has been associated with higher rates of turnover and decreased productivity
contributing to an impending nursing and physician shortage.[5]

The purpose of this systematic review was to examine factors associated with
burnout of nurses in the United States. Only studies that used the 22-item Maslach
Burnout Inventory-Health Services Survey (MBI-HSS), in its entirety, to measure
burnout were included in this analysis.

Instrument Description

The MBI-HSS is the most commonly used instrument to measure burnout among
health care providers.[13] The MBI-HSS is a norm-referenced 22-item, 7-point Likert-
type instrument (0 indicates the feeling of burnout "never" happens to 6 indicating
the feeling of burnout happens "every day") with 3 subscales: emotional exhaustion
(EE) (9 items), depersonalization (DP) (5 items), and personal accomplishment (PA)
(8 items). Maslach and Jackson[14] have defined these variables as follows:

- Emotional exhaustion: measures feelings of being emotionally overextended and
  exhausted by one's work.
- Depersonalization: measures an unfeeling and impersonal response toward recipients of one's service, care treatment, or instruction.
- Personal accomplishment: measures feelings of competence and successful
  achievement in one's work.

Scores for each of the subscales are calculated separately and not combined into a
composite score. The 3 subscales measure different dimensions of burnout and are
not highly correlated as to constitute a single construct.[15] Researchers have used
the EE scale as a proxy to measure burnout. Maslach and colleagues do not support
the use of a single subscale, as they propose that burnout is more than fatigue or
exhaustion and that it includes high levels of depersonalization and low levels of personal accomplishment.[15]

Maslach and colleagues recommend scoring the scale using 1 of 2 methods.[15] The
first method is to simply add the responses to the items for each scale and use the sum
of the scaled score, resulting in a range between 0 to 54 for EE, 0 to 30 for depuson-
alization, and 0 to 48 for personal accomplishment. In the second scoring method the
total score for the scale is divided by the number of items on the scale to determine the

mean score. For example, a mean score of 5.5 would indicate a respondent felt emotionally exhausted several times a week but not every day.

The MBI-HSS is the original and most widely used version of the MBI. Designed for professionals in the human services, the psychometric rigor of the MBI-HSS has been well documented in the literature and has been recognized as a psychometrically sound instrument.[15–17] The MBI-HSS has been administered to nurses and other health care providers around the world and is available in multiple languages.

METHODS
Design

A systematic review was conducted following the Preferred Reporting Items for Systematic Reviews and Meta-Analysis guidelines.[18] A systematic process was used to select relevant studies, extract and analyze data, and rate the quality of the studies.

Search Methods

A librarian performed systematic searches using the following databases: PubMed/ Medline, CINAHL, PsycInfo, ProQuest, Embase, Cochrane, ERIC, and TRIP. The databases were searched from January 2000 to December 2019, and only peer-reviewed scholarly journal articles were included. The search terms included (burnout OR burn-out OR burn out) AND Maslach AND nurse. A Boolean strategy using the operators AND and OR enhanced the searches and ensured a comprehensive search was completed.

Inclusion Criteria

Studies were included in the systematic review if they met the following inclusion criteria: (1) the study was a quantitative analysis of empirical data using the MBI-HSS, (2) all 3 subscales of the 22-item MBI-HSS were used, (3) the sample consisted of registered nurses, (4) sample size for the study was reported, (5) the study was published between 2000 and 2019, (6) study setting was in the United States, and (7) the study was published in English. Studies before 2000 were not included because care delivery approaches were changing and improvements in the efficiency of care were being adapted. In addition, studies conducted outside of the United States were excluded because the health care systems and practice environments are different in other countries as compared with the United States.

Study Screening

Fig. 1 provides a summary of the literature search and study selection process. The search of electronic databases yielded 6533 titles and abstracts. Following the removal of duplicates, non-English articles, and conference abstracts or presentations, there were 2391 titles/abstracts screened for inclusion. The titles and abstracts of articles were independently screened by 2 reviewers on the research team to determine if the inclusion criteria were met. Any disagreements were discussed, until consensus was reached. Articles were excluded only if both reviewers agreed that the inclusion criteria were not met.

There were 927 full-text articles screened for eligibility. Each article was screened by 2 independent reviewers from the research team. Any disagreements were resolved by a third reviewer. After the screening of articles was completed, 16 studies met the inclusion criteria and were included in the systematic review. The most common reasons for exclusion of studies from the systematic review were the following: (1) studies did not use all 22-items on the MBI-HSS, (2) studies only included physicians, and (3) studies not being conducted in the United States. There were 280 studies that

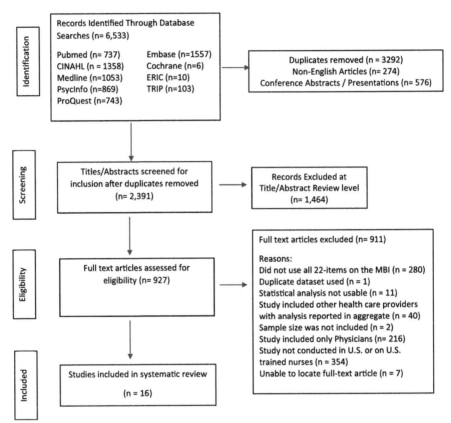

Fig. 1. Preferred Reporting Items for Systematic Reviews and Meta-Analysis (PRISMA) flow diagram describing selection of publications.

did not use the complete version of the MBI-HSS. Most of these studies only used the EE subscale or a combination of the EE and DP or PA scales. According to guidance from Maslach and colleagues they do not support only using 1 or 2 of the subscales to measure burnout.[15] They believe all 3 subscales should be used to ensure adequate representation of the construct of burnout and to maintain consistency and allow comparability with prior research findings. Therefore, only studies using all 3 subscales were included in this review.

Data Extraction Process

The following data were extracted from each of the studies: authors, year of publication, sample size and demographics, study setting, country where the study was conducted, study design, data collection method, psychometric properties of the instrument, and variables correlating with burnout. The data extraction was conducted by 2 independent reviewers and all disagreements were resolved by a third reviewer.

Quality Assessment

The methodological quality of each study meeting the full inclusion criteria was assessed by 2 members of the research team using a quality rating instrument adapted from previously published systematic reviews.[19–24] The adapted instrument assesses 4 categories of each study: research design, sample, measurement, and statistical analysis. The instrument includes 13 criteria; 12 of the criteria were scored 0 = not met and 1 = met, and 1 criterion related to the measurement of burnout was scored with 2 = objective observation, 1 = self-report, and 0 = not reported. The use of self-report presents an increased threat to construct validity, so a greater weight was applied to that criterion. The range of total quality points was 0 to 14: all studies with scores 0 to 4 were considered low quality, 5 to 9 were considered medium quality, 10 to 14 were considered high quality. Any discrepancies noted between the 2 reviewers were discussed, and consensus was reached.

RESULTS
Characteristics of the Studies

Table 1 provides a summary of the characteristics of the 16 studies included in the systematic review. All of the studies used the 22-item HHS version of the MBI. The research designs for these studies were descriptive correlational (n = 13), mixed methods (n = 2) and quasi-experimental (n = 1). All of the descriptive correlational studies used cross-sectional survey designs that were either mailed or distributed in person to the participants. The quasi-experimental study used a single group pre-post design to examine burnout before and after the implementation of a Developmental Care Partner Program. Both of the studies using a mixed methods design used a survey and semistructured qualitative interviews to collect data.

The sample sizes ranged from 25 to 2837 nurses who worked in various settings in the United States. The study by Card and colleagues included a national sample of perianesthesia nurses that consisted of 2837 nurses.[27] There were 9 studies that had a sample of 100 or less nurses. The remaining 6 studies had sample sizes between 101 and 888 nurses.

The scoring for the MBI-HSS varied across the studies in the review. There were 10 studies that used the first scoring method described in the instrument description section and provided cutoff scores for low, moderate, and high levels of burnout. Lanz and colleagues used the second scoring method and reported means for the subscale scores.[31] Finally, 5 studies reported bivariate correlations but did not identify the scoring methodology used to obtain the correlations.

Quality Reviews

Of the 16 studies that were evaluated for quality, the total scores ranged from 7 to 11. There were 4 studies of high quality, 12 studies of medium quality, and 0 studies with low quality (**Table 1**). As described in the methods section, the methodological quality of each study was assessed, and **Table 2** provides an aggregate summary of the quality assessment. Across all of the studies there were 3 major weaknesses related to sample size justification, reporting of reliability coefficients, and use of a theoretic/conceptual model to guide the study.

Sample size justification was not reported in any of the studies, and this was not surprising because most of the studies used a convenience sample and a descriptive correlational design. Convenience sampling is needed in many of these types of studies because researchers are targeting specific groups of nurses who work in specific specialties to assess their level of burnout. Reliability coefficients were only reported in 5 of the 16 studies, and 3 of the 13 studies reported using a theoretic/conceptual framework to guide their study.

A major strength of these studies was noted in each quality assessment category. All the sixteen studies reported the study design, clearly defined study variables,

Table 1
Study characteristics

First Author/Year of Publication	Purpose	Setting and Sample	Study Design	Findings	Study Quality
Adwan,[25] 2014	Explore relationships between pediatric nurses' grief experiences resulting from patient deaths with burnout and job satisfaction.	Large midwestern academic medical center—120 pediatric RNs	Descriptive correlational	Grief was significantly correlated with burnout (positive) and job satisfaction (negative). RNs reported significantly higher EE when primary patients died and higher guilt if patients were young.	High
Browning et al,[26] 2006	Examine the impact of personality characteristics, specifically, cognitive adaptation disposition, on expectations-burnout relationship.	Multisite—36 states and different specialties—341 RNs	Descriptive correlational	Cognitive adaptation predicted fewer unmet expectations of control, which was associated with lower burnout. Lower expectations of control were associated with high EE and DP and low PA. Optimism and self-esteem were associated with lower burnout (lower EE, lower DP, and higher PA) regardless of perceived expectations of control.	High

| Card et al,[27] 2019 | Investigate the prevalence and factors affecting job burnout in a national sample of perianesthesia nurses. | National Sample of 2837 perianesthesia nurses | Descriptive correlational | There was a lower incidence of burnout in nurses older than 40 y. Lower burnout was associated with regular participation in physical, creative, and mindfulness hobbies. Burned out nurses perceived a lack of advancement opportunities and organizational investment as well as poorer physical and mental health. EE had the highest score on the burnout inventory. | Medium |
| Clubbs et al,[28] 2019 | Evaluate the feasibility of a developmental care partner program in a level III NICU and determine its relationship with nurse burnout and infant infection rates. | Midwest community hospital NICU—25 RNs | Pre-/postquasiexperimental study | Postintervention (DCP program) nurses reported significantly lower EE scores. The DP score was lower but not significant, and the PA score remained unchanged. The DCP program could help reduce EE and DP in nurses. | Medium |

(continued on next page)

Table 1
(continued)

First Author/Year of Publication	Purpose	Setting and Sample	Study Design	Findings	Study Quality
Davis et al,[29] 2013	Investigate differences in burnout among oncology nurses by type of work setting, coping strategies, and job satisfaction.	Metropolitan cancer center—74 oncology nurses	Descriptive correlational	Younger nurses (<40 years old) reported a lower level of EE as compared with older nurses (>40 year old). RNs working in an outpatient setting reported a higher level of EE as compared with RNs working in inpatient settings. Highly significant correlations were noted among job satisfaction and EE and among job satisfaction and intent to leave oncology. Spirituality and relationships with coworkers were the 2 most frequently used coping strategies when dealing with burnout.	High
Gallagher & Gormley,[30] 2009	Examine relationships among nurse stress, burnout, and perceptions of support systems.	Academic, Pediatric Medical Center in the Midwest—30 bone marrow transplant nurses	Descriptive correlational	>70% of nurses perceived high levels of EE, 33% moderate levels of DP, and 50% high levels of PA. 90% of RNs felt that support systems were in place, but >50% were undecided about the helpfulness of these systems.	Medium

Author, Year	Purpose	Sample/Setting	Design	Findings	Quality
Gueritault-Chalvin et al,[9] 2000	Determine which psychological coping skills are related to burnout in health care professionals working with HIV/AIDS patients.	Center for AIDS intervention research—445 nurses	Descriptive correlational/path analysis	There was a positive association between workload and burnout scores. External coping was positively related to burnout, and internal coping was negatively associated with burnout. Path analysis showed workload, age, locus of control, and external and internal coping were predictors of burnout independently or after controlling for specific variables.	Medium
Jameson & Bowen,[10] 2020	Describe the relationship between the school nurse practice environment, school nurses' levels of burnout, and perceived sources of work stress.	New Jersey State School Nurses Association—100 school nurses	Descriptive correlational	Burnout was significantly associated with all areas of work life. Workload made the strongest unique contribution to explaining EE. School districts with satisfactory work environments reported lower rates of burnout. School nurses reported moderate levels of EE, low levels of DP, and high levels of PA.	Medium

(continued on next page)

Table 1
(continued)

First Author/Year of Publication	Purpose	Setting and Sample	Study Design	Findings	Study Quality
Lanz & Bruk-Lee,[31] 2017	Examine the relative effects of interpersonal conflict and workload on job outcomes (turnover intentions, burnout, injuries) and if resilience moderates the indirect effects of conflict and workload on job outcomes.	Sample of US nurses—97 RNs	Descriptive/correlational 2-wave design	Interpersonal conflict at work predicted turnover intentions and burnout as measured by EE, DP, and PA in RNs. Increased workload predicted an increase in self-reported nurse injuries.	High
Mealer et al,[32] 2012	Determine whether resilience was associated with lower prevalence of symptoms of posttraumatic stress disorder and burnout.	Sample of ICU RNs from American Association of Critical-Care Nurses membership list—744 ICU RNs	Descriptive/Correlational	There was a high rate of burnout in the sample of RNs: 61% of RNs reported having EE; 44% for DP; and 50% for lack of PA. The presence of higher resilience scores in RNs was associated with the absence of burnout syndrome, a diagnosis of posttraumatic stress disorder, and symptoms of depression and/or anxiety.	Medium

Meltzer & Missak-Huckabay,[33] 2004	Determine the relationship between critical care nurses' perceptions of futile care and its effect on burnout.	Two hospitals in Southern California—60 critical care RNs	Descriptive/Correlational	Nurses encounters with moral distress situations involving futile care was positively related to EE. Younger RNs had increased feelings of DP as compared with nurses older than 46 years. Nurses with a bachelor's degree or higher experienced more painful feelings of futility as compared with associate degree RNs.	Medium
Messmer et al,[34] 2011	Examine intent to stay and the relationship between work satisfaction and burnout.	Pediatric specialty hospital in South Florida—33 RNs	Descriptive/Correlational	Significant correlation reported between work satisfaction and burnout. The higher the perceived work satisfaction, the lower the burnout rate.	Medium
Muir & Keim-Malpass, 2020	Examine burnout score changes and drivers of burnout while assessing the feasibility of a mindfulness intervention program for Emergency Department RNs and Patient Care Technicians (PCTs).	Emergency department RNs and PCTs in an urban level 1 trauma center in Virginia. Time 1–26 RNs and Time 2–20 RNs	Mixed methods pre-/ post-intervention design	At time 1 RNs had higher scores in EE and DP as compared with PCTs. At time 2 RNs had significant decreases in EE and increases in PA. Results suggest that RNs are important clinicians, who work in high stress and unpredictable environments, RNs should be targeted for burnout interventions given the noted score changes from time 1 to time 2.	Medium

(continued on next page)

Table 1
(continued)

First Author/Year of Publication	Purpose	Setting and Sample	Study Design	Findings	Study Quality
Peery,[36] 2010	Examine the relationship between caring and burnout in RNs.	North Carolina RNs—888 RNs	Descriptive/Correlational	The carative factors of respectful deference for the other, assurance of human presence combined with attentiveness to others' experiences, professional knowledge and skill, and positive connectedness were all predictors of PA. Because nurses care more through connecting with patients and developing trusting relationships they experience lower levels of EE and DP.	Medium
Rainbow & Steege,[37] 2019	Explore the transition to nursing practice experience of first- and second-career RNs.	Midwestern Academic Medical Center—122 RNs	Mixed methods	Burnout and presenteeism prevalence were thematic findings in the qualitative interviews, and there were differences in burnout rates in the quantitative data. There was a large effect size in levels of DP across time points.	Medium

| | | | | Presenteeism and burnout are related, as they both decrease nurse performance and engagement at work. Both first and second career nurses were aware of the prevalence of these issues and were taking steps to avoid becoming burned out. | |
| Russell,[38] 2016 | Identify perceptions of burnout among oncology nurses. | University of Pittsburgh Medical Center—61 RNs | Descriptive/Correlational | Burnout was at a moderate level for EE, DP, and PA in this sample of RNs. When higher levels of support and care are demanded from patients or family members burnout increases. Burnout was lower in nurses with >10 y of experience. Nurses strongly believe that burnout has a negative impact on the care they provide. Collaboration among staff and resources and supplies decreased nurse burnout levels. | Medium |

Abbreviations: HIV, human immunodeficiency virus; NICU, neonatal intensive care unit; RN, registered nurses.

Table 2
Summary of quality assessment

Summary of Quality Assessment (n = 16)		
	Number of Studies	
Design	Yes	No
Was the study design reported?	16	0
Were key study variables clearly defined?	16	0
Sample		
Was sample size justified?	0	16
Was the sample drawn from more than one site?	9	7
Was the response rate more than 30%?	11	5
Was the sampling approach described?	16	0
Measurement		
Was the reliability of each subscale reported for the study sample?	5	11
Was the reliability of each subscale >.70?	7	9
Was burnout measured using a valid instrument?	16	0
Was the outcome of burnout observed rather than self-reported? (2 points = observed; 1 point = self-report; 0 points = not reported)	0	16
Was a theoretic model or framework used for guidance?	3	13
Statistical Analysis		
Were outliers managed/controlled?	8	8
If multiple outcomes were analyzed, were correlations analyzed?	15	1

clearly described the sampling approach, used a valid instrument to measure burnout, and provided correlations when multiple outcomes were analyzed. All of the studies used a self-report approach to data collection, except 2 studies that used qualitative inquiries and made comparisons with the quantitative self-report data. Although all 16 studies received a "no" for the observation versus self-report item, this is not an unexpected finding because studies that did not use the MBI-HSS, which is a self-report instrument, were excluded.

Factors Associated with Burnout

Workload is a primary stressor in the work environment. Workload is a complex concept to measure and one that must include contextual and organizational characteristics germane to the nursing work environment. There were 3 studies that concluded workload correlated with EE, DP, PA, and predicted burnout.[9,10,31] Jameson and Bowen indicated that workload made the strongest unique contribution to explaining EE (B = −0.43, $P < .000$), while controlling for all other variables.[10] In addition, they found that DP (r = −0.31, $P < .01$) was negatively correlated with workload, and nurses who perceived high levels of PA experienced lower levels of burnout. Lanz and Bruk-Lee tested a model examining the effects of workload on burnout and found that there was a significant indirect effect of workload on EE (0.47), DP (0.34), and PA (−0.20); all confidence intervals for the indirect effects excluded zero.[31] As workload increased, EE and DP increased, but as PA increased, workload decreased. Another interesting finding in this study was that injuries were significantly predicted by increased workload (effect = 0.55, $P = .04$). Each of the burnout subscales accounted for a significant amount of variance in the model predicting injuries at work.

There is evidence from 3 studies that job satisfaction was associated with increased burnout.[25,29,34] Adwan reported that job satisfaction was negatively correlated with EE ($r = -0.46$, $P < .001$) and DP ($r = -0.36$, $P < .001$) and positively correlated with PA ($r = 0.24$, $P = .009$). In addition, the grief experience of nurses was positively associated with EE ($r = 0.38$, $P < .001$) and DP ($r = 0.19$, $P = .04$) and negatively correlated with PA ($r = -0.24$, $P = .009$).[25] Davis and colleagues found that there were highly significant correlations ($r = 0.67$, $P < .001$) between job satisfaction and EE.[29] Messmer and colleagues reported a strong, positive significant correlation between work satisfaction and burnout ($r = -0.68$, $P < .001$); the higher the perceived work satisfaction, the lower the burnout rate. In a regression model, work satisfaction scores accounted for 42% of the variance in burnout.[34]

A healthy nursing work environment is a critical factor in the care that is provided to our patients and the satisfaction of the nurses. Evidence from 9 different studies in this review indicate that a healthy work environment is linked to increased satisfaction and reduced burnout.[10,27–29,31,34,35,37,38] Although only one study included in this review measured work environment satisfaction,[34] there were 8 other studies that implemented different measures or programs that were expected to improve social and physical aspects of the work environment and decrease burnout.[10,27–29,31,35,37,38] Messmer and colleagues correlated scores from the Nursing Work Index, instrument used to measure satisfaction with the work environment, and the MBI-HSS, finding a strong, negative correlation ($r = -0.68$, $P < .001$). Overall, the findings in this study showed that the higher the perceived work satisfaction, the lower the burnout in nurses.[34] There were social and work-based stressors identified by Lanz and Bruk-Lee,[31] in a study of hospital-based nurses, that predicted burnout. Specifically, interpersonal conflict at work was significantly correlated with EE ($r = .44$, $P < .01$), DP ($r = .50$, $P < .01$), and PA ($r = -.31$, $P < .01$) and in the multiple regression model was the only variable that explained significantly unique variance in EE (B = .37, $P < .001$), DP (B = .45, $P < .001$), and PA (B = $-.37$, $P < .001$). In a study by Card and colleagues[27] they reported a strong relationship among nurses who were currently experiencing burnout and having a negative perception of the work environment ($P < .001$). In addition, EE was the most frequent response to burnout followed by PA and DP.

Evidence from 5 studies indicated that age significantly predicts burnout.[9,26,27,29,33] In each of these studies the overall indication is that as age increases, burnout decreases. In 2 of the studies younger nurses had significantly higher DP scores as compared with older nurses.[27,33] One study reported that younger nurses had significantly higher PA scores as compared with older nurses (>40 year old).[27] EE was reported to be higher in younger nurses as compared with nurses who were older than 40 years.[27,29] There were 2 studies that analyzed years of experience and found that nurses with more years of experience reported decreased EE ($r = -0.57$, $P < .05$) and DP ($r = -0.34$, $P < .05$) and increased PA ($r = 0.49$, $P < .05$).[30,38]

Another interesting characteristic was the relationship between control and burnout. Three studies found that perceived loss of control was associated with greater burnout.[9,26,27] Browning and colleagues used a regression model and reported that nurses' lower current expectations of control (greater unmet) were significantly related to higher levels of EE (B = -0.40, $P < .001$) and DP (B = -0.28, $P < .001$) and lower levels of PA (B = 0.24, $P < .001$).[26] Internal and external locus of control were measured in one study.[9] Internal locus of control was defined as individuals who believe they have the ability to influence their environment, and external control referred to those individuals who perceive events as being under the control of luck, chance, or fate (ie, factors external to themselves). The study reported one composite score for locus of control. The results of this study showed that locus of control accounted for 4.5% of the variance in burnout scores. In the path analysis model locus of control had a direct effect on burnout (B = −0.13, P < .01), indicating that increased influence over the environment was associated with lower levels of burnout.

There were several studies who identified coping strategies to assist nurses in decreasing burnout.[9,26–29,32,33,35,36] Mindfulness was investigated in 2 of the studies,[27,35] and there was a significant negative association with burnout. Mealer and colleagues reported that a higher level of resilience in nursing staff was associated with decreased burnout, depression, and anxiety.[32] Spirituality was used by nurses as a coping strategy, and this reduced stress and burnout.[29,33]

DISCUSSION

This systematic review aimed to identify research that measured burnout in US nurses with the intent of discovering factors associated with burnout. The studies included in the review were only those that used the 22-item MBI-HSS to measure burnout. The key factors that were associated with burnout and/or the 3 subscales of the MBI-HSS were workload, job satisfaction, work environment, interpersonal conflict, control, age, and years of experience. The findings from this study were consistent with research that has been reported on burnout in nurses and the association with variables such as high workload, job satisfaction, lack of support, and work environment.[7,8]

Healthy work environments are effective in attracting and retaining nurses and are associated with decreased burnout, job satisfaction, and improved patient outcomes.[39–42] Most of the interventions identified, such as mindfulness or social and work-based stressors, in this review were targeting individuals or small groups of individuals. More research is needed to identify strategies and target specific organizational factors that affect the hospital system and will make improvements across work environments throughout the organization. Hospitals that achieve Magnet designation are associated with healthier work environments, improved nurse outcomes, and reduced burnout.[43]

Workload is a critical factor associated with nurse burnout. Based on this review, interventions that allow nurses to increase their PA and reduce EE and DP will counteract other variables that contribute to high levels of burnout. Workload will vary by specialty types, but if adequate staffing is available to meet the patient demands, there is evidence that this will improve productivity and patient outcomes while decreasing nurse burnout.[44]

Most of the studies in this review lacked a theoretic or a conceptual approach. The absence of a conceptual model does not permit a comprehensive understanding of burnout in the workplace. Maslach and Jackson described the concept of burnout and developed a measurement instrument that is now dominating health professions research as the leading instrument to measure burnout.[14,15] Over the last few decades, there have been many changes in the health care environment, but one constant has been nurse burnout and its implications on the individual and the organization. It is imperative that nurse researchers consider a new definition and conceptualization of burnout that is more aligned with current workforce needs and organizational structures.

Empirical studies need to move beyond the descriptive correlational designs that rarely report relationships between more than 1 or 2 variables. The use of quasi-experimental and/or experimental research to enable researchers to assert causality and generalizability in relation to their findings as well as obtain a better understanding of burnout in nurses at the individual and organizational levels is needed. Longitudinal designs will allow researchers to follow individuals over time to get a better understanding of the work-related variables contributing to burnout. The descriptive correlational designs have provided sufficient evidence to indicate that burnout has negative implications on the work environment, staff, and the organization.

The MBI-HSS has been established as a reliable and valid instrument to measure burnout across many professions.[15] The 3 dimensions of the MBI-HSS (EE, DP, and PA) are all separate subscales and do not result in a composite score for burnout. The studies in this review had varying cut-offs for high, medium, and low levels of burnout, and some studies combined scores to develop a composite score for burnout. The inconsistency with which burnout dimensions are measured is problematic and does not allow for fair comparisons across studies. There were several studies (n = 280) that were excluded from this review because they only used 1 or 2 dimensions of burnout, and the guidance from Maslach and colleagues is that all 3 dimensions are to be used, as they all provide a different aspect of burnout. Finally, there is no definitive score from the MBI-HSS that "proves" an individual is burned out.[15]

SUMMARY

The available evidence from all studies in this review supports a positive relationship with burnout, and factors such as a healthy work environment, manageable workload, collaborative relationships with coworkers and leadership, job satisfaction, support through spirituality, greater connectedness with the nurse and the patient, and adequate resources may decrease burnout. The development of a new conceptual model, a new instrument, or significant revisions to the existing MBI-HSS instrument and its scoring is needed to ensure better alignment with the current practice environments. Finally, as nursing leaders we need a reliable instrument to allow us to recognize burnout, ameliorate the symptoms, and promote a healthy work environment for all staff.

CLINICS CARE POINTS

- Administrators must support nurses at the bedside with needed resources for reducing burnout.
- Healthy work environments are associated with more satisfied nurses and increased quality of care at the bedside.
- Increased workloads are correlated with decreased satisfaction and increased EE of nurses at the bedside, which indirectly has a negative effect on patient care.
- Designing a mechanism to all nurses to engage in coping strategies such as mindfulness training, will reduce burnout in bedside nurses.

DISCLOSURE

The authors have nothing to disclose.

REFERENCES

1. Mehta S, Machado F, Kwizera A, et al. COVID-19: A heavy toll on health-care workers. Lancet Respir Med 2021;9(3):226–8.

2. Lasater KB, Aiken LH, Sloane DM, et al. Chronic hospital nurse understaffing meets COVID-19: an observational study. BMJ Qual Saf 2021;30(8):639–47.

3. Rosa WE, Schlak AE, Rushton CH. A blueprint for leadership during COVID-19. Nurs Manage 2020;51(8):29–34.

4. World Health Organization. Burn-out an "occupational phenomenon": International Classification of Diseases. 2019. Available at: https://www.who.int/news/item/28-05-2019-burn-out-an-occupational-phenomenon-international-classification-of-diseases. Accessed June, 2021.

5. Reith TP. Burnout in United States Healthcare Professionals: a narrative review. Cureus 2018;10(12):e3681.

6. Swensen S, Strongwater S, Mohta NS. Leadership survey: immunization against burnout. Nurs Manag 2018;4(2):1–14.

7. Dall'Ora C, Ball J, Reinius M, et al. Burnout in nursing: a theoretical review. Hum Resour Health 2020;18(41):1–17.

8. Dyrbye LN, Shanafelt TD, Johnson PO, et al. A cross-sectional study exploring the relationship between burnout, absenteeism, and job performance among American nurses. BMC Nurs 2019;18(57):1–8.

9. Gueritault-Chalvin V, Kalichman SC, Demi A, et al. Work-related stress and occupational burnout in AIDS caregivers: test of a coping model with nurses providing AIDS care. AIDS Care 2000;12(2):149–61. References marked with an asterisk (*) indicate studies included in the systematic review.

10. Jameson BE, Bowen F. Use of the worklife and levels of burnout surveys to assess the school nurse work environment. J Sch Nurs 2020;36(4):272–82. References marked with an asterisk (*) indicate studies included in the systematic review.

11. Liu Y, Aungsuroch Y. Factors influencing nurse -assessed quality nursing care: A cross-sectional study in hospitals. J Adv Nurs 2018;74(4):935–45.

12. Carayon P, Gurses AP. Nursing workload and patient safety—a human factors engineering perspective. In: Hughes RG, editor. Patient safety and quality: an evidence-based handbook for nurses. Rockville (MD): Agency for Healthcare Research and Quality (US); 2008. p. 203–16. Available at. https://www.ncbi.nlm.nih.gov/books/NBK2657/.

13. Trockel M, Bohman B, Lesure E, et al. A Brief instrument to assess both burnout and professional fulfillment in physicians: reliability and validity, including correlation with self-reported medical errors, in a sample of resident and practicing physicians. Acad Psychiatry 2018;42(1):11–24.

14. Maslach C, Jackson SE. The measurement of experienced burnout. J Organ Behav 1981;2:99–113.

15. Maslach C, Jackson SE, Leiter MP. Maslach Burnout Inventory Manual. 4th edition. Menlo Park, CA: Mind Garden, Inc; 2018. Available at: https://www.mindgarden.com/117-maslach-burnout-inventory-mbi.

16. Beckstead JW. Confirmatory factor analysis of the Maslach Burnout Inventory among Florida nurses. Int J Nurs Stud 2002;39:785–92.

17. Poghosyan L, Aiken LH, Sloane DM. Factor structure of the Maslach Burnout Inventory: An analysis of data from large scale cross-sectional surveys of nurses from eight countries. Int J Nurs Stud 2009;46(7):894–902.

18. Moher D, Liberati A, Tetzlaff J, et al. The PRISMA Group. Preferred reporting items for systematic reviews and meta-analyses: the PRISMA statement. PLoS Med 2009;6(7):e1000097.

19. Cummings GG, Estabrooks CA. The effects of hospital restructuring including layoffs on nurses who remained employed: a systematic review of impact. Int J Sociol Soc Policy 2003;23(8–9):8–53.

20. Cummings GG, Lee H, MacGregor T, et al. Factors contributing to nursing leadership: a systematic review. J Health Serv Res Policy 2008;13(4):240–8.

21. Cummings GG, MacGregor T, Davey M, et al. Leadership styles and outcome patterns for the nursing workforce and work environment: A systematic review. Int J Nurs Stud 2010;47(3):363–85.

22. Cummings GG, Tate K, Lee S, et al. Leadership styles and outcome patterns for the nursing workforce and work environment: a systematic review. Int J Nurs Stud 2018;85:19–60.

23. Estabrooks CA, Floyd JA, Scott-Findlay S, et al. Individual determinants of research utilization: a systematic review. J Adv Nurs 2003;43(5):506–20.

24. Wong CA, Cummings GG. The relationship between nursing leadership and patient outcomes: A systematic review. J Nurs Manag 2007;15(5):508–21.

25. Adwan JZ. Pediatric nurses' grief experience, burnout and job satisfaction. J Pediatr Nurs 2014;29:329–36. References marked with an asterisk (*) indicate studies included in the systematic review.

26. Browning L, Ryan CS, Greenberg MS, et al. Effects of cognitive adaptation on the expectation-burnout relationship among nurses. J Behav Med 2006;29(2): 139–50. References marked with an asterisk (*) indicate studies included in the systematic review.

27. Card EB, Hyman SA, Wells N, et al. Burnout and resiliency in perianesthesia nurses: Findings and recommendations from a national study of members of the American Society of PeriAnesthesia Nurses. J Perianesth Nurs 2019;34(6): 1130–45. References marked with an asterisk (*) indicate studies included in the systematic review.

28. Clubbs BH, Barnette AR, Gray N, et al. A community hospital NICU developmental care partner program: Fe-asibility and association with decreased nurse burnout without increased infant infection rates. Adv Neonatal Care 2019;19(4): 311–20. References marked with an asterisk (*) indicate studies included in the systematic review.

29. Davis S, Lind BK, Sorensen C. A comparison of burnout among oncology nurses working In adult and pediatric inpatient and outpatient settings. Oncol Nurs Forum 2013;40(4):E303–11. References marked with an asterisk (*) indicate studies included in the systematic review.

30. Gallagher R, Gormley DK. Perceptions of stress, burnout, and support systems in pediatric bone marrow transplantation nursing. Clin J Oncol Nurs 2009;13(6): 681–5. References marked with an asterisk (*) indicate studies included in the systematic review.

31. Lanz JJ, Bruk-Lee V. Resilience as a moderator of the indirect effects of conflict and workload on job outcomes among nurses. J Adv Nurs 2017;73:2973–86. References marked with an asterisk (*) indicate studies included in the systematic review.

32. Mealer M, Jones J, Newman J, et al. The presence of resilience is associated with a healthier psychological profile in intensive care unit (ICU) nurses: Results of a national survey. Int J Nurs Stud 2012;49:292–9. References marked with an asterisk (*) indicate studies included in the systematic review.

33. Meltzer LS, Missak-Huckabay L. Critical care nurses' perceptions of futile care and its effect on burnout. Am J Crit Care 2004;13(3):202–8. References marked with an asterisk (*) indicate studies included in the systematic review.

34. Messmer PR, Bragg J, Williams PD. Support programs for new graduates in pediatric nursing. J Contin Educ Nurs 2011;42(4):182–92. References marked with an asterisk (*) indicate studies included in the systematic review.

35. Muir KJ, Keim-Malpass J. The emergency resiliency initiative: A pilot mindfulness intervention program. J Holist Nurs 2020;38(2):205–20.

36. Peery AI. Caring and burnout in registered nurses: What's the connection? Int J Hum Caring 2010;14(2):53–60. References marked with an asterisk (*) indicate studies included in the systematic review.

37. Rainbow JG, Steege LM. Transition to practice experiences of first- and second-career nurses: A mixed-methods study. J Clin Nurs 2019;28:1193–204. References marked with an asterisk (*) indicate studies included in the systematic review.

38. Russell K. Perceptions of burnout, its prevention, and its effect on patient care as described by oncology nurses in the hospital setting. Oncol Nurs Forum 2016; 43(1):103–9. References marked with an asterisk (*) indicate studies included in the systematic review.

39. American Association of Critical-Care Nurses. AACN standards for establishing and sustaining healthy work environments: A journey to excellence (Executive Summary 2nd, edition) 2016. Available at: http://www.aacn.org/wd/hwe/docs/execsum2016.pdf. Accessed March 3, 2021.

40. Carthon B, Margo J, Hatfield L, et al. System-level improvements in work environments lead to lower nurse burnout and higher patient satisfaction. J Nurs Care Qual 2021;36(1):7–13.

41. Copanitsanou P, Fotos N, Brokalaki H. Effects of work environment on patient and nurse outcomes. Br J Nurs 2017;26(3):172–6.

42. Havaei F, Astivia OL, MacPhee M. The impact of workplace violence on medical-surgical nurses' health outcome: a moderated medication model of work environment conditions and burnout using secondary data. Int J Nurs Stud 2020; 109:1–9.

43. Lasater KB, Germack HD, Small DS, et al. Hospitals known for nursing excellence perform better on value-based purchasing measures. Policy Polit Nurs Pract. 2016;17(4):177–86.

44. Perez-Francisco DH, Duarte-Climents G, Rosario-Melian JM, et al. Influence of workload on primary care nurses' health and burnout, patients' safety, and quality of care: Integrative review. Healthcare 2020;8(12):1–14.

Early Career Burnout in Nursing

Marcos Gayol, EdD, MSN, MPH, RN, CNE, CPH*, Tracy Lookingbill, DNP, MSN, RN

KEYWORDS

- Early career nurses • Nursing workforce • Burnout • Stress
- Maslach Burnout Inventory

KEY POINTS

- The prevalence of burnout within the early career nursing population can be influenced by a variety of contributing stress factors.
- Burnout has no official definition though the prevalence of burnout is impacting the nursing workforce.
- The consequences of burnout affect the health and well-being of nurses, patients, patient care, and more broadly, the organization.

INTRODUCTION

Early career burnout among nurses is a complex and consequential state of well-being impacting the nursing workforce. Among health care workers in the United States (US), burnout syndrome is a widely recognized problem with increasing emphasis in recent years.[1] Stress, overwhelmingness, and anxiety are associated with burnout syndrome among those who provide care to patient populations associated specifically with stressful work environments.[2] Among U.S. nurses, approximately 35% to 45% experience professional burnout directly related to chronic work-related stressors. A primary factor relating to early career nurse burnout is workload with an estimated 30% of all new graduates leaving the profession with less than 1 year of experience. Workplace resources available to nurses do not align with the workforce demands resulting in mental, physical, and ultimately emotional exhaustion.[1,3,4] Early career nurses are essential to the future of the nursing workforce. Early career nurses who maintain optimal mental and physical health show increased satisfaction and commitment to organizations.[5]

New graduates and early career nurses report experiencing moral distress due to ethical conflicts with workplace relationships and a loss of empowerment within the role. Health care settings are associated with unpredictable environments, competing

Aspen University, School of Nursing and Health Sciences, 1660 South Albion Street, Suite 225, Denver, CO 80222, USA
* Corresponding author.
E-mail address: marcos.gayol@aspen.edu

Nurs Clin N Am 57 (2022) 21–28
https://doi.org/10.1016/j.cnur.2021.11.002
0029-6465/22/© 2021 Elsevier Inc. All rights reserved.
nursing.theclinics.com

demands, and complex decision-making resulting in an imbalance of nurse well-being and coping mechanisms.[6,7] Burnout among early career nurses is identified through various chronic stressors within the nursing profession. Identified stressors are often associated specifically with people-focused careers among health care professionals, social work, and law enforcement. Research supports nurse leaders are essential for recognizing environmental work stressors among new nurse graduates and promoting self-care among nurses.

As a consequence of nurse burnout, individuals may experience deterioration of psychological and physiological health. Prolonged exposure to excessive workplace demands can impact a nurse's response to environmental demands and cogitative function. Collaboration and communication are often nonexistent and lack appeal among early career nurses. The American Nurses Association (ANA) Year of the Health Nurse Campaign recognized the need to create improved work environments and strategies to increase resilience among nurses.[8] Although health care organizations are impacted by early career burnout among nurses as well as patient outcomes, research for well-being and reconginzation of burnout is lacking.[3,9]

HISTORY

Current research discusses consequences related to early career burnout. Research indicates that unwanted professional progression is common among nurses who experience burnout. Early career nurses who experience burnout are less likely to engage in leadership roles, disengage in work, and ultimately leave the profession. Within the health care setting, nurse burnout has a relationship to higher mortality rates and lower patient satisfaction scores with suboptimal care for patients.[10] The National Academy of Medicine (NAM) recognizes burnout as significant emotional exhaustion, decreased personal accomplishment, and increased depersonalization. Among the lack of social support within the health care setting, non-supportive work environments are identified as contributing factors. Important considerations of early burnout among nurses indicate that each nurse may be affected differently.[11]

Nurses who provide care to specialized populations have a higher prevalence of burnout. A reported estimate of nurses caring for patients who are critically ill experience burnout at a rate of 50%. Oncology nurses (38%) and palliative care (35%) additionally experience higher rates of burnout.[12] New graduates often experience culture shock as they transition from the academic setting into real-world health care settings. The academic setting prepared the nurse graduate as a competent achievement-oriented setting without the complexities related to a hierarchical system with dominant behaviors. As a result of the dramatic shift between student to nurse, transitional dissatisfaction in early nursing practice can quickly escalate leading to internal conflict and moral distress.[4]

The profession of nursing has been recognized as a significantly stressful profession based on the nature of the roles and exposure to ongoing conflict within health care systems. External stress indicators are recognized as contributing factors for early career burnout. Within the academic setting, rigorous requirements of entry into practice and professional demands are challenging for early career nurses to meet. The unpredictable balance of professional responsibilities and family commitments impacts mental health and well-being.[13] Early career nurses may experience high levels of stress and vulnerability. In critical care units, new nurse graduates are reported to have a significant increase in intention to leave the role reporting stress as the most significant reason.[5]

CONSIDERATIONS

Health care systems are facing current nursing shortages which are anticipated to worsen in the coming years.[14] The multidimensional considerations associated with burnout lead to increased stress on individual nurses and institutions. Negative working conditions have consequential effects on role commitment, attitudes, healthy coping techniques, lower quality of care, miscommunications, decreased staff retention, and overall job performance. Nurses report chronic stress and overwhelmingness leading to professional inadequacy result in an overall detachment from the role. As a direct result of nurse burnout, institutions face specific unit issues as absenteeism has a strong relationship to burnout leading to social and economic consequences. The loss of workforce at the unit level leads to a decrease in productivity, lower morale, and more frequent use of overtime within the current employee pool.[7]

High workforce turnover rates within health care systems aggravate an already stressed system. Early career nurses have an estimated turnover rate between 17% and 50% globally within the first 12 months of graduation. Consequentially, leading to poor patient outcomes and economic impacts.[15] Hospital systems have implemented residency programs to increase self-efficacy and provide an internal support structure throughout the initial stages of novice practice.[16] Offering early career nurses the opportunity to explore various specialties within the hospital system allow the new graduate to feel in control of their decision with clinical preferences and create a sense of fulfillment, accomplishment, and belongingness.

The correlations between early career burnout among nurses and poor patient outcomes in health care systems are directly connected. Research studies correlate poor patient outcomes with stressful working environments leading to increased mortality and adverse events among patients. However, work environments associated with safe, structured, and collaborative work environments supported improved patient outcomes. An example of a positive work setting reported by nurses with favorable patient outcomes includes magnet-designated hospitals. Magnet-designated hospitals focus on nurse role empowerment, evidenced-based practice, and innovation created through collaboration.[14]

BURNOUT DISCUSSION

A critical component of early career turnover and early career termination is due to burnout. Among new graduates, many report a loss of empowerment over decision-making and role dissatisfaction.[16] Feelings of inexperience coupled with high-stress environments are foundational to burnout.[4] The transition between academics and real-world practice often lack the appropriate preparedness as newly graduated nurses enter professional practice. The consequences of burnout among early career nurses have a direct relationship to increased workplace turnover, emotional distress, decreased work performance, physical illness, and negative attitudes among nurses.

Health care systems are motivated to increase understanding of burnout to determine predictors of early career nurse burnout and potential indicators to improve retention and employee satisfaction. Effects of nurse burnout have shown a direct relationship between poor quality of care and safety among patient populations.[3,4] Identifiable constraints are often motivated by extrinsic factors in health care systems related to inequitable workforce distributions. Nurses have challenges navigating institutional and hierarchy imbalances ultimately impacting nurse decision making and patient outcomes. Emotional and physical health, communication, and coping among nurses are directly linked to early career burnout within the nursing profession.[14]

The term burnout is often aligned with the term moral distress. Andrew Jameton defined "moral distress" as constrained actions within the nursing profession when a challenging situation creates internal conflict between ethics and external obstacles. Moral distress is significantly linked to job satisfaction and retention.[17] Although moral distress is directly linked to burnout in many health care professions, nurses are more prone to experience this specific type of distress. Current research indicates the role of a novice nurse in the work setting are influenced by internal and external stressors. Factors associated with a lack of confidence, new responsibilities, and a misaligned transition from academica to the work setting contribute to burnout.[18] Additionally, workplace violence has a significant impact among nurses leading to burnout.[19] Research suggests coping strategies such as social support and self-efficacy can have a positive outcome when managing early career burnout in nurses.[3]

While burnout has no medical condition classification and does not have an official definition within the nursing profession, health care worker burnout syndrome was first described by Herbert Freudenberger in 1974.[20,21] Freudenberger described burnout as an individual's state of irritability and an inability to cope with stress, leading workers to exhaustion, fatigue, and an overwhelming feeling of defeat. Specifically, Freudenberger described burnout relating to work demands, factors, and environments.

Later in the 1980s, Susan Jackson and Christina Maslach further explored the psychological concepts of burnout among health care workers and suggested that burnout was a syndrome encompassed by 3 main components that include emotional exhaustion, depersonalization, and personal accomplishment which are defined in **Fig. 1**.[22]

TOOL TO MEASURE BURNOUT

Maslach and Jackson created the *Maslach Burnout Inventory* (MBI). From the original MBI concepts, a refinement of the 22-item tool called the Maslach Burnout Inventory-Human Services Survey (MBI-HHS) was developed. The MBI-HHS assesses the 3 subscales listed in **Fig. 1** and is a valid and reliable assessment tool widely used to measure burnout frequency in health care workers and has been used to measure burnout among nurses.

Maslach and Jackson[22] defined the 3 main components as follows:

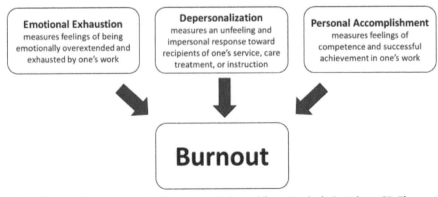

Fig. 1. Three main components of burnout. (*Adapted from* Maslach C, Jackson SE. The measurement of experienced burnout. J Organ Behav. 1981; 2: 99-113. doi.org/10.1002/job.4030020205.)

- Emotional exhaustion (9-items): measures feelings of being emotionally overextended and exhausted by one's work.
- Depersonalization (5-items): measures an unfeeling and impersonal response toward recipients of one's service, care treatment, or instruction.
- Personal accomplishment (8-items): measures feelings of competence and successful achievement in one's work.

Of the 22 items within the MBI-HHS, 9 items address emotional exhaustion to measure fatigue related to work or work outcomes and associated feelings of emotional overextension. Five of the 22 items measure depersonalization which is an unfeeling response by which the individual seems detached and unempathetic toward work. Eight of the 22 items measure personal accomplishment issues which surround feelings of discouragement related to lack of self-perceived diminishing sense of accomplishment or contribution.[22]

Burnout Profiles

Maslach, Jackson, and Leiter[23] label profiles as: "Overextended, Disengaged and Ineffective" and describe patterns of emotional exhaustion, depersonalization, and personal achievement across the 3 profiles. The *overextended* profile presents with high levels of exhaustion, the *disengaged* profile showroom presents with higher levels of depersonalization, and *cynicism* and the *ineffective* profile shows low levels of efficacy. Understanding the various profiles within an organization is crucial when designing initiatives and interventions to combat burnout.

High workload and work frequency directly impact emotional exhaustion for individuals presenting in the overextended profile. For the disengaged profile, the workload is not as much the main issue as a feeling of disconnection or unfeeling toward their work, organization, or team that contributes to the central focus of depersonalization. Alternately, the lack of supportive relationships and environments influence the individual's sense of personal accomplishment with the ineffective profile.

Contributing Factors

Considering burnout is a complex state of being tired, discouraged, and detached, the reasons underpinning burnout are equally as complex. Early career nurses experience a wide variety of organizational-level factors that may contribute to burnout associated with work stress which includes high workload, incentivized work and overtime, low work satisfaction, long work schedules, and poor work orientation and environment. Similarly, early career nurses may also experience individual factors that can contribute to burnout including lack of self-care and underutilization of resilience strategies.

Work stress is a primary contributing factor to burnout and is a complicated concept because multiple issues may occur simultaneously within an organization, at the institutional, unit, or team level. Workload is associated with high stress and has been a continuous and recurring issue within the nursing profession. Nurse personnel shortages[24] and budgetary restrictions can impact the assignment of patients and nurse-patient ratios, and new nurses often have no control over the assignment or the ratio of patients. Institutions often market and monetarily incentivize positions within nursing specialties areas that requirement caring for patients of high acuity within emergency departments and critical care units.[5] Nursing units often monetarily incentivize overtime work and new nurses are enticed by the additional income, which leads to working extra hours and adding to their work stressors.

Because new nurses lack extensive career experience to care for high-acuity patients, immersive training is required. However, comprehensive training is inconsistent throughout the US. Poor work orientation can contribute to work stress as a result of feeling underprepared for work responsibilities and expectations. Poor social support, nonsupportive work environments, and lack of socialization to and with the team create unintentional consequences for new nurses leading to conflicts, unprofessional behavior, and poorer work relationships. Factors indicated at the individual level include unhealthy coping methods for stress management, poor sleep patterns, and poor self-care practices.[13]

RECOMMENDATIONS

To mitigate the circumstances and factors contributing to burnout, organizations need to design interventions to address various aspects of the work stress experienced by early career nurses. Capping overtime and reassessing reasonable staffing ratios are the first step organization should take to ensure higher job satisfaction and lower emotional exhaustion among new nurses. Planned, structured, consistent, and supported orientation programs for new nurses have proven to increase retention of new graduates and extended nurse residency programs are a way to socialize new nurses into their role while supporting the development of professional relationships, shared sense of identity, personalization, and integration within the organization and team.[25] Extended orientations and nurse residencies with mentorship also assist the new graduate's transition from a reward system in academia to one of expert practice and personal accomplishment. The extended orientation will positively impact a new nurse's sense of competence and confidence in the care they provide.

To foster a supportive culture, institutional commitment to wellness is an essential part of preemptively addressing burnout. Wellness programs, such as the STAR (Stress, Trauma, and Resilience) program offered by the organization have also been recognized to improve the mental health and well-being of new nurses and have had a positive impact on the retention of those who participate in the program.[26] The Department of Defense's Patient Safety Program in partnership with the Agency for Healthcare Research and Quality's Team Strategies and Tools to Enhance Performance and Patient Safety (Team-STEPPS) is a training tool developed to assist organizations to reduce traits that contribute to poor communication and poor team dynamics.[26] Training on proven self-care practices is a needed focus to provide new nurses with strategies to be more mindful and intentional with specific activities with regards to coping and managing work-related stress.[5]

CLINICS CARE POINTS

- When determining staffing ratios and workload, organizations should hire a sufficient amount of staff to avoid overtime usage and calculate ratios based on acuity and workload rather than solely the number of patients.
- When orienting new nurses, focus an extended period of mentorship that is patient-focused and measures personalization of the new nurse's engagement with coworkers and the recipients of their work.
- When considering the creation and implementation of wellness and self-care training and programs, focus on feelings of competence, and successful achievement in one's work.

SUMMARY

The future of the nursing workforce is dependent on early career nurses' successful integration in the nursing profession. Burnout prevalence among the early career nurse population is a complex issue negatively affecting the retention of nurses, and impacting the wellbeing of new nurses. In recent years, a greater emphasis has been placed on the contributing factors to burnout[1] and the largest part of the responsibility to correct these stress factors can be addressed at the organizational, unit, team, and individual levels. Work-related stress, anxiety, and sense of overload are associated with approximately 35% to 45% of burnout experienced by nurses in the United States and 30% of early career nurses leave the profession with less than a year of service.[3]

Organizational initiatives, services, and programs like extended orientations, nurse residencies, STAR, Team-STEPPS, and self-care training can positively impact job satisfaction and the emotional, mental, and physical well-being of early career nurses as well as their commitment to organizations and the nursing profession.[5]

DISCLOSURE

The authors have nothing to disclose.

REFERENCES

1. Denat Y, Gokce S, Gungor H, et al. Relationship of anxiety and burnout with extrasystoles in critical care nurses in Turkey. Pak J Med Sci 2016;32(1):196–200.
2. Schooley B, Hikmet N, Tarcan M, et al. Comparing burnout across emergency physicians, nurses, technicians, and health information technicians working for the same organization. Medicine 2016;95(10):1–6.
3. Diehl E, Rieger S, Letzel S, et al. The relationship between workload and burnout among nurses: The buffering role of personal, social and organizational resources. PLoS ONE 2021;16(1):1–17.
4. Bong HE. Understanding moral distress: how to decrease turnover rates of new graduate pediatric nurses. Pediatr Nurs 2019;45(3):109–14.
5. Feddeh SA, Darawad MW. Correlates to work-related stress of newly-graduated nurses in critical care units. Int J Caring Sci 2020;13(1):507–16.
6. Vincent L, Brindley P, Highfield J, et al. Burnout syndrome in UK intensive care unit staff: Data from all three Burnout Syndrome domains and across professional groups, genders and ages. J Intensive Care Soc 2019;20(4):363–8.
7. Salvagioni DAJ, Melanda FN, Mesas AE, et al. Physical, psychological and occupational consequences of job burnout: A systematic review of prospective studies. PLoS ONE 2017;12(10):1–29.
8. Borg Card E, Hyman S, Wells N, et al. Burnout and resiliency in paranesthesia nurses; Findings and recommendations from a national study of members of the American Society of PeriAnesthesia nurses. J PeriAnesthesia Nurs 2019; 34(6):1130–45.
9. Gates R, Musick D, Greenwald M, et al. Evaluation the burnout-thriving index in a multidisciplinary cohort at a large academic medical center. South Med J 2019; 112(4):199–204.
10. Dyrbye L, Shanafelt D, Johnson P, et al. A cross-sectional study exploring the relationship between burnout, absenteeism, and job performance among American nurses. BMC Nurs 2019;18(1):1–8.
11. Kurosaka A. Prevention strategies to cope with nurse burnout in nephrology settings. Nephrol Nurs J 2020;47(6):539–63.

12. Higgins JT, Okoli C, Otachi J, et al. Factors associated with burnout in trauma nurses. J Trauma Nurs 2020;27(6):319–23.
13. Allen HK, Barrall AL, Vincent KB, et al. Stress and burnout among graduate students: moderation by sleep duration and quality. Int J Behav Med 2021; 28(1):21–8.
14. Van Bogaert P, Peremans L, Van Heusden D, et al. Predictors of burnout, work engagement and nurse reported job outcomes and quality of care: a mixed method study. BMC Nurs 2017;18:1–14.
15. Mills J, Chamberlain-Salaun J, Harrison H, et al. Retaining early career registered nurses: a case study. BMC Nurs 2016;15:1–6.
16. Kuokkanen L, Leino-Kilpi H, Numminen O, et al. Newly graduated nurses' empowerment regarding professional competence and other work-related factors. BMC Nurs 2016;15:1–8.
17. Fourie C. Moral distress and moral conflict in clinical ethics. Bioethics 2015; 29(2):91–7.
18. Van Wijlen J. Healing the healer: a caring science approach to moral distress in new graduate nurses. Int J Hum Caring 2017;21(1):15–9.
19. Duan X, Ni X, Shi L, et al. The impact of workplace violence on job satisfaction, job burnout, and turnover intention: the mediating role of social support. Health Qual Life Outcomes 2019;17(1):1–10.
20. Freudenberger H. Staff burn-out. J Social Issues 1974;30(1):159–65.
21. Freudenberger H. The staff burn-out syndrome in alternative institutions. Psychotherapy: Theor Res Pract 1975;12(1):73–82.
22. Maslach C, Jackson SE. The measurement of experienced burnout. J Occup Behav 1981;2:99–113.
23. Maslach C, Jackson SE, Leiter MP. Maslach burnout inventory manual. 4th edition. Mind Garden, Inc; 2018. Available at: https://www.mindgarden.com/117-maslach-burnout-inventory-mbi.
24. The American Association of Colleges of Nursing. Nursing shortage. AACN. 2019. Available at: https://www.aacnnursing.org/Portals/42/News/Factsheets/Nursing-Shortage-Factsheet.pdf.
25. Brook J, Aitken L, MacLaren J, et al. An intervention to decrease burnout and increase retention of early career nurses: a mixed methods study of acceptability and feasibility. BMC Nurs 2021;20:1–12.
26. Wu T, Fox D, Stokes C, et al. Work-related stress and intention to quit in newly graduated nurses. Nurse Education Today 2012;32(6):669–74.

Factors Associated with Burnout in the United States Versus International Nurses

Debra Sullivan, PhD, MSN, RN, CNE, COI[a],*,
Kathleen M. White, PhD, RN, NEA-BC[b],
Christine Frazer, PhD, CNS, CNE[a,b]

KEYWORDS

- Nursing burnout • MBI • Intention to leave • Nurse satisfaction • Job stress
- Workplace violence

KEY POINTS

- Nurse burnout is an ongoing serious problem in the United States and internationally.
- Factors associated with nurse burnout are significant problems for nurses, patients, and organizations.
- There are interventions aimed at reducing nurse burnout that individuals and organizations should consider.

INTRODUCTION

Burnout is a global health care workforce problem. In the past few years, the growing prevalence of burnout syndrome among health care workers has gained attention. It has been a significant issue for the nursing profession for years, and the nursing literature is replete with studies that report burnout is a common problem among nurses both in the United States and internationally. Nursing outcomes have been affected by this problem and have been researched. In this article, the factors associated with nurse burnout are researched in the US compared with international findings.

In 2019, the World Health Organization (WHO) declared burnout an "occupational phenomenon."[1] Burnout is included in the 11th Revision of the International Classification of Diseases as an occupational phenomenon, not a medical condition.[1] It is designated QD85 burnout and further described as "problems associated with employment or unemployment."[1] Burn out is defined as a syndrome resulting from

[a] College of Nursing, Walden University, 100 Washington Avenue South, Suite 1210, Minneapolis, MN 55401, USA; [b] Emerita Johns Hopkins University, School of Nursing, 525 N. Wolfe Street, Baltimore, MD 21205, USA
* Corresponding author. 1581 Cunningham Road, Readyville, TN 37149.
E-mail address: Debra.sullivan@mail.waldenu.edu

Nurs Clin N Am 57 (2022) 29–51
https://doi.org/10.1016/j.cnur.2021.11.003
0029-6465/22/© 2021 Elsevier Inc. All rights reserved.

chronic workplace stress that has not been successfully managed. It is characterized by 3 dimensions:

- Feelings of energy depletion or exhaustion;
- Increased mental distance from one's job or feelings of negativism or cynicism related to one's job; and
- Reduced professional efficacy.

The term "burnout" was first used by an American psychologist, Herbert Freudenberger, who defined burnout as "to fail, wear out, or become exhausted by making excessive demands on energy, strength, or resources."[2] He described burnout as a consequence of dealing with constant stress in the helping professions.[2] The concept of burnout was further developed by Maslach and Jackson, who characterized burnout in 3 domains: emotional exhaustion (EE), depersonalization (DP), and a diminished sense of personal accomplishment (PA).[3]

Burnout is a Serious Problem in the United States and Worldwide

In the fall of 2020, Maslach and colleagues collaborated with the Harvard Business Review to gather data in 46 countries to understand the extent of burnout around the world.[4] Eighty-nine percent of respondents said their work life was getting worse; 85% said their well-being had declined; 56% said their job demands had increased; and 62% of the people who were struggling to manage their workloads had experienced burnout "often" or "extremely often" in the previous 3 months. Only 21% of respondents rated their well-being as "good," with 2% rating it as "excellent." The survey respondents scored high on exhaustion and cynicism, 2 predictors of burnout.[4]

Burnout is a severe workplace problem today, and the problem started well before the Covid-19 pandemic hit. Many workers were already experiencing high levels of burnout; the pandemic simply compounded the already escalating problem.

Maslach Burnout Inventory—United States and Worldwide

Since the Maslach Burnout Inventory (MBI) was first published in 1981, several new versions of the MBI have been developed for use with different groups and different settings. The Maslach Burnout Inventory-Human Services Survey (MBI-HSS) is the version used to measure burnout in health care professionals.[4] It was originally developed in English and has been used to measure the presence of burnout in nurses and other health care providers in many English-speaking countries, including the United States, England, Scotland, Australia, and New Zealand. The MBI-HSS has been translated into more than 45 languages. The recent systematic review conducted in 2022 by Zangaro and colleagues[5] reviewed studies from more than 33 countries, at least 6 English speaking countries, and 27 others. Researchers in countries who are attempting to study burnout for the first time need to consider the translation and how it will affect the validity and reliability of the translated version of the instrument. A list of the languages that all versions of the MBI have been translated into is available at Mind Tools Web site: https://www.mindgarden.com/117-maslach-burnout-inventory-mbi#horizontalTab3. New translations are added all the time to the Web site.

The MBI is the gold standard in measuring burnout.[6] It has been used and revised since 1981,[3] and the psychometric properties have been established in several studies.[7-11] The MBI is also used to measure burnout in nurses in the United States and internationally, as it has been translated in many languages.[4] The following discussion will report on findings in the literature on factors associated with nurse burnout as measured by the MBI, comparing the US with international studies.

Factors Associated with Nurse Burnout

Factors associated with nurse burnout can result in adverse job characteristics, such as negative nurse outcomes. To test hypotheses about whether there is an association between these factors and nurse burnout, tools such as these have been correlated with the MBI measurements. Because this has been done both internationally and in the United States, the results of these studies are compared in the following discussion.

In the systematic review by Zangaro and colleagues[5] there were 927 articles from the years 2000 to 2019, which were first filtered for titles and abstracts that included the entire MBI-HSS and were written in English. Maslach[3] and colleagues have stated that all 3 subscales should be used to ensure appropriate application of the construct of burnout. For this reason, Zangaro and colleagues[5] only included studies in the systematic review in the United States and used the entire MBI where all 3 subscales were administered. In this section, the investigators went a step further and screened for factors associated with nurse burnout and the country of origin. The following information was also gathered in order to compare the studies, types of instruments to measure the factors that were correlated with the MBI, and the conclusions of their research. The most common factors were found to be "Intention to Leave," Job Stress," Job Satisfaction," and Workplace Violence." These factors as they related to nurse burnout will be reported on in the following literature review.

Intention to Leave

The nursing shortage has been an ongoing problem for many years. In a report by the WHO, the International Council of Nurses and Nursing Now,[12] there is global shortfall of 5.9 million nurses with greatest need in countries in Africa, South East Asia, and Eastern Mediterranean region, as well as parts of Latin America. As a result of the nursing shortage, nurse retention is important due to the cost of nurse turnover, which in 2018 in the United States was estimated at $52,100 per position.[13] In an attempt to mitigate nurse turnover, studies have been done to determine reasons nurses leave their employment.

In screening the articles in the Zangaro and colleagues'[5] systematic review, researchers have hypothesized that nursing burnout may be related to a nurse's intention to leave their job. Eleven articles were found that looked at the nurses intention to leave their job, and of those, 11[14–24] were done in countries outside the United States, with surprisingly none in the United States. Only one of the articles did not find a relationship between intention to leave and nurse burnout.[19] In **Table 1**, the instruments that were used to measure intention to leave, the article citation, country of origin, and a short summary of the reported findings are listed.

Recommendations that were made to mitigate nursing burnout and decrease intention to leave included interventions to improve the work environment, staffing allocations, increase income, strengthening group cohesion, training in conflict management, as well as broader training opportunities.[16]

In summary, the overwhelming majority of the international studies reviewed using the MBI to measure burnout in nurses and various tools to measure intention to leave found a significant positive relationship between burnout and the intention to leave their job; this would indicate that interventions to lower nurse burnout could decrease the intention to leave outcome and be beneficial in retaining nurses.

Job Stress

In nursing, the relationship between job stress and burnout has been recognized for decades.[30] Liao and colleagues[31] found that higher levels of job-induced stress

Table 1
Intention to leave

Tool Used to Measure Intention to Leave	Article Reference	Country	Findings
Turnover Intention Scale (from the Questionnaire for the Perception and Assessment of Labor; van Veldhoven & Meijman,[25] 1994)	Vermeir et al,[14] 2018	Belgium	Researchers found a low number of high intention to leave or 6.6% with low burnout scores of 3%
A question asked on the questionnaire for example, "do you intend to leave your current job?"	Lorenz & Sabino,[15] 2018	Brazil	MBI showed 28.0% of nurses with emotional exhaustion, with a weak correlation coefficient 0.34 with intention of leaving current work and nursing
	Jiang et al,[16] 2017 Jourdain & Chênevert,[17] 2010 Leiter et al,[18] 2009	China Canada Canada	Found high levels of burnout associated with intention to leave
	Arikan et al,[19] 2007	Turkey	25.8% of nurses working in dialysis intended to leave the nursing profession in the near future but had low burnout scores
	Arslan & Kocaman,[20] 2016	Turkey	30% of all nurses intended to leave their work place and all had high burnout scores
Practice Environment Scale of the Nursing Work Index[26–28]	Bruyneel et al,[21] 2017	Belgium	Turnover intention only partially mediated by burnout
	Langerlund et al,[22] 2015	Sweden	About one-third of all RNs intended to leave their workplace within the next year and with higher burnout scores
Intent to Stay Scale[29]	Meng et al,[23] 2015	China	Burnout had a negative effect on intent to stay
Personal Accomplishment Subscale Intention to Quit/Change Questionnaire[24]	Pienaar & Bester,[24] 2011	South Africa	Respondents with the highest levels of motional exhaustion and depersonalization and the lowest levels of personal accomplishment displayed a higher degree of intention to quit/change

Table 2 Job stress			
Tool Used to Measure Job Stressors	**Article Reference**	**Country**	**Findings**
Nurse Job Stressors Inventory[44]	Luan et al[33]	China	Positive correlations between job stress and burnout among senior nurses ($r = 0.554$, $P < .01$) than head nurses ($r = 0.426$, $P < .01$)
Nurse Stress Checklist[45]	Liao et al[34]	Taiwan	Job-induced stress was a significant factor affecting emotional exhaustion ($\beta = 0.608$, $P < .001$) and depersonalization ($\beta = 2.439$, $P < .001$)
Nursing Stress Inventory[46]	Khamisa et al[35]	South Africa	Job stressors are significantly associated with burnout; patient care (OR 2.24, 95% CI 1.94–2.59), staff issues (OR 4.18 95% CI 2.93–5.96), lack of support (OR 4.37 95% CI 2.89–6.62), overtime (OR 2.12, 95% CI 1.78–2.53)
Nursing Stress Scale[46]	Hayes et al[36]	Australia	In dialysis, nurses' high levels of emotional exhaustion were linked to stress of the job rather than due to decreased job satisfaction
Nursing Stress Scale[47]	Portero de la Cruz et al[37]	Spain	A significant and positive relation was found between the professionals' global stress level and their emotional exhaustion and depersonalization
Leiden Quality of Work Questionnaire[48]	Adriaenssens et al[38]	Nether-lands	Changes over time in job characteristics (JDCS: job demands, control, and social support) were significantly related to emotional exhaustion
Mental Health Professional Stress Scale[49]	McTiernan et al[39]	Ireland	Moderate stress with low burnout scores

(*continued on next page*)

Table 2
(continued)

Tool Used to Measure Job Stressors	Article Reference	Country	Findings
Job Stressors Scale[50]	Tuna et al[40]	Turkey	Significant relationship was established between subdimensions of job stress level and burnout level
Work-Related Strain Inventory[51]	Arikan et al[19]	Australia	Reported decreased job stress and burnout, but no relationship reported
Job-Related Stress Questionnaire—self-designed	Jaracz et al[41]	Poland	Significant effect of stress on burnout
	Jamal et al[42]	Canada	Job stress was significantly correlated with overall burnout and its 3 dimensions
	Assadi et al[43]	Iran	Nurses suffered from high occupational burnout in stressful jobs

Abbreviations: CI, confidence interval; OR, odds ratio.

resulted in higher levels of occupational burnout. Occupational stress is defined by the WHO as "work demands and pressures that are not matched to their knowledge and abilities and which challenge their ability to cope."[32] Job stress can have a negative effect on the nurses' ability to solve problems and quality of care for patients.[33]

There were 14 articles retrieved that reported on job stress, as it relates to burnout.[19,34–43] Twelve research articles found a significant positive relationship with job stress and burnout; as job stress increases, burnout increases and in the reverse as job stress decreases, burnout decreases.[34–43] There were 2 studies that fell outside these findings: one in Ireland[40] that found nurses with moderate stress and low burnout scores and the second one from Australia[19] that found decreased job stress and burnout, but no relationship was reported. In **Table 2**, the instruments that were used to measure job stress, the article reference, country of origin, and a short summary of the reported findings are listed.

Recommendations found in the reviewed articles to mitigate job stress that leads to burnout were strategies to reduce burnout and stress management.[52] Also important are ways to support nurse autonomy, control over work environment, nurse recognition, ensure adequate workload, increase work efficiency, and professional relationships.[38] In summary, most of the international studies reviewed using the MBI to measure burnout and various tools to measure job stress in nurses found a significant positive relationship between burnout and job stress. Job stress could be seen as a predictor of burnout, and this would indicate that interventions to lower job stress would also lower nurse burnout.

Job Satisfaction

Globally, the nursing profession prevalence of burnout and job dissatisfaction is high.[53] To explore job dissatisfaction and burnout among nurses, Aiken and

Table 3
Factors tied to job satisfaction

Factor	Article	Findings
Core components to job satisfaction	• Abushaikha & Saca-Hazboun,[57] 2009 • Hayes et al,[52] 2010 • Hayes et al,[58] 2015 • Nwafor et al,[59] 2015 • Utrianen & Kyngas,[60] 2009 • van der Doef et al,[61] 2012 • Vermeir et al,[14] 2018 • Zangara & Soeken,[62] 2007 • Arikan et al,[19] 2007 • Happel & Koehn,[63] 2011 • Khamisa et al,[35] 2016 • Liu et al,[64] 2015 • Ozden et al,[65] 2013 • Palazoglu & Koc,[66] 2019 • Roulin et al,[67] 2014 • Vermeir et al,[68] 2018	Throughout several decades, research studies sought to deepen the awareness of nurse job satisfaction and lessen the gravity of job dissatisfaction, thereby decreasing associated nurse burnout. A review of the research literature identified multiple attributes as significant core components to nurse job satisfaction, such as autonomy, interpersonal relationship, and patient care.[52,57,58,59,60,61,62] Factors such as self-concept, interprofessional teamwork, communication, management support, good relationship with patients, praise and acknowledgment about quality of care provided, and balanced work-family life link to nursing job satisfaction.[15,20,36,52,58,59,60,65,66,67,68]
Practice environment	• Alharbi et al,[55] 2016 • Palazoglu & Koc,[66] 2019 • Liu et al,[64] 2015 • Palazoglu & Koc,[66] 2019 • Hayes et al,[52] 2010 • van der Doef et al,[61] 2012	Nurses in emergency department/clinic,[55,56] critical care (pediatric ICU, adult ICU,[55,64,66] in-center acute hemolysis units). Hayes et al[52] report significant job dissatisfaction and a higher incidence of burnout. Attributing to burnout and a decrease in job satisfaction in these specialized areas were sources of stress such as overwhelmed with time pressure, limited resources, physical working conditions, fatigue, and patient deaths[52,55,61,66]
Demographic Factors	• Palazoglu & Koc,[66] 2019 • Akman et al,[69] 2016	*Age:* Palazoglu & Koc[66] note that nurses older than 40 y were significantly more satisfied ($P = .003$) than those younger than 40 y. Furthermore, Akman et al[69] report age (mean = 28.95; SD = 6; range 18–55; $\beta = -0.296$) and job satisfaction ($\beta = 0.431$) significantly ($P < .001$) contribute to burnout levels. Specifically, an increase in age of a nurse job satisfaction contributes to lower burnout level
	• Hayes et al,[52] 2010 • Liu et al,[64] 2015	*Experience:* Hayes et al[52] findings report nurses working 20 y or more had the highest satisfaction score (mean = 3.60, SD = 0.69) and those who worked less than a year were less satisfied (mean = 3.12, SD = 0.54). Although no significant difference related to age, Liu et al's[64] analysis results identify significant differences in job

(continued on next page)

Table 3 (continued)		
Factor	**Article**	**Findings**
		satisfaction among nurses with different years of work experience (P = .030). Specifically, nurses with <5 y or 10–19 y of experience report higher job satisfaction compared with nurses with 5–9 or more than 20 y of experience. Moreover, years of work experience significantly predicted job satisfaction. Those with 10–20 y were 4.484 times more likely to be satisfied in comparison to nurses with more than 20 y (CI = 1.195–16.830, P = .026).

Abbreviations: CI, confidence interval; ICU, intensive care unit; SD, standard deviation.

colleagues[54] surveyed nurses and patients in 12 countries in Europe and the United States. Concerning burnout, results showed that a significant proportion of nurses in every country reported high nurse burnout.[54]

Research findings note a correlation between job satisfaction and burnout, indicating one factor precedes the other.[35,55] In **Table 3**, practice environment and demographics as they relate to nurse burnout are summarized.

From Zangaro and colleagues'[5] systematic review, researchers hypothesized that nurse burnout might be associated with nurse job satisfaction. Specific to nurses and job satisfaction or dissatisfaction, 22 research articles were found, with only one research article from the United States.[56] Most articles were from Turkey (5), Australia (4), and Africa (3). All but 6 studies[14,37,57,63,69,70] reported a relationship between nurse job satisfaction and burnout. **Table 4** presents these instruments, research article of reference, country of origin surrounding the research, and a brief summary of the findings.

Recommendations shared within the literature aim to positively affect nurse job satisfaction at the individual, group, and organizational level and, in turn, decrease burnout. In **Table 5**, these recommendations are reviewed.

In summary, significant predictors to job satisfaction occur at the individual, group, and organizational level.[67] Burnout is shown to be a significant problem in nurses who experience job dissatisfaction. Job dissatisfaction has significant outcomes on nurse burnout, which in turn affects not only the health care workforce (ie, retention, turnover, absenteeism), influences the health of nurses, and also affects outcomes associated with the patient population served (ie, patient satisfaction, patient safety).[52,55,57,69]

Workplace Violence

Workplace violence (WPV) is a serious problem facing health care delivery systems and health care workers (HCW) globally.[83] Research findings show a connection between interpersonal conflict and burnout; therefore, emotions are triggers that can potentially lead to WPV between employees.[83] The American Nurses Association[84] reports violence against HCW is at "epic proportions." Perpetrators of violence in health care facilities are most often patients and relatives, although employee-to-employee

Table 4
Job satisfaction[74]

Tool Used to Measure Job Satisfaction	Article Reference	Country	Findings
The Leiden Quality of Work Life Questionnaire for Nurses (LQELQ—nurse's version)[74]	van der Doef & Maes,[27] 2015	East Africa—Tanzania, Kenya, and Uganda	Results of MBI indicated East African nurses are burned out. The nurses working in public hospital experience a lower job satisfaction compared with nurses in private hospitals. Multiple regression analysis showed a high job satisfaction is related to better staffing (β = 0.14, P < .05), higher supervisor support (β = 0.21, P < .0001), better interdepartmental cooperation (β = 0.13, P < .05), and adequacy of financial reward (β = 0.18, P <.01).
Index of Work Satisfaction (IWS)[75]	Hayes et al,[36] 2015	Australia	Quantitative findings revealed years of work (>20) had the highest overall mean job satisfaction score (M = 3.60, SD = 0.69) compared with nurses who worked the shortest amount of time. Greatest job satisfaction obtained from professional status (M = 5.35, SD = 0.89), then interactions in the workplace (M = 4.88, SD = 1.05), and autonomy (M = 4.84, SD = 1.08). EE significantly associated with lower overall job satisfaction (r = −0.56, P < .01). Qualitative findings report an association between nurse job satisfaction and ability to provide "good" care, forming close relationships with patients, and in their role, feeling successful, a sense of pride and proficient.
IWS—Part B of instrument[75]	Adwan,[56] 2014	United States	IWS assesses nurse responses on job satisfaction (strong agreement to strong disagreement) in 6 areas (pay, autonomy, task requirements, organizational policies, interaction, and professional status). MBI burnout level moderate EE and PA, low DP. Correlation among the MBI & IWS total scores are EE (r = −0.464, P < .001), PA (r = 0.238, P = .009), DP (r = −0.358, P <.001).

(continued on next page)

Table 4
(continued)

Tool Used to Measure Job Satisfaction	Article Reference	Country	Findings
Job Satisfaction Survey (JSS)[76]	Alharbi et al,[55] 2012	Saudi Arabia	Increases in perceptions of DP were correlated with a decrease in satisfaction with supervision ($r = -0.24$, $P = .002$), co-workers ($r = -0.16$, $P = .048$), and nature of work ($r = -0.25$, $P = .002$). Increased EE is correlated with reduced satisfaction with contingent rewards ($r = -0.34$, $P < .001$), operating conditions ($r = -0.24$, $P = .003$), and communication ($r = -0.29$, $P < .001$). PA was moderately positively associated with supervision ($r = 0.31$, $P < .001$), co-workers ($r = 0.24$, $P = .003$), and nature of work ($r = 0.43$, $P < .001$). Results indicate an increase in PA correlates with a lower satisfaction with fringe benefits, contingent rewards, and operating conditions ($r = -0.23$, $P = .004$; $r = -0.18$, $P = .028$; $r = -0.30$, $P < .001$, respectively).
	Khamisa et al,[35] 2016	South Africa	EE is most significantly associated with job satisfaction (OR = 2.37, 95% CI 2.13–2.63). Job satisfaction with promotion is most significantly associated with burnout (OR = 1.14, 95% CI 1.05–1.23). Job satisfaction with supervision, operating conditions, contingent rewards, pay, fringe benefits, and coworkers are not associated with nurse burnout.
Job Satisfaction Scale of the Nurse Stress Index	Pinikahana & Happell,[70] 2004	Australia	Rural psychiatric nurses are satisfied with current work situation (66.1%), level of involvement in decision-making (65.4%), and degree of job support they receive (61.7%). A significant proportion of rural psychiatric nurses (70.8%) scored low in burnout. No significant relation of job satisfaction burnout.
Minnesota Satisfaction Questionnaire (MSQ)[77]	Palazoglu & Koc,[66] 2019	Turkey	A higher level of nurse burnout was associated with a decrease in job satisfaction ($r = -0.335$, $P < .001$). Mean general satisfaction scores differed significantly according to age ($P = .003$), love of occupation ($P \leq .001$), quality of work-life balance ($P \leq .001$), and satisfaction at work institution ($P \leq .001$). A weak and negative correlation between MBI and MSQ noted ($r = -0.335$, $P < .001$).
	Topbas et al,[71] 2019	Turkey	Negative association between MSQ scores and DP ($r = -0.427$, $P < .05$) and EE ($r = -0.564$, $P < .05$). Thus, as job satisfaction increased, emotional exhaustion (EE) and depersonalization (DP) scores decreased.

Source	Country	Findings
Akman et al,[69] 2016	Turkey	Among pediatric nurses, job satisfaction significantly ($P < .001$) explained burnout level experienced ($B = 11.985$, $SE = 1.813$, $\beta = 0.431$). A medium level relation between intrinsic, extrinsic, and general job satisfaction and EE ($r = 0.58$; 0.58; and 0.63, respectively) and DP (0.47; 0.36; and 0.46, respectively) was reported. A low-level relationship between PA, internal ($r = 0.21$, $P < .001$), and general satisfaction ($r = 0.19$, $P < .001$).
Nwafor et al,[59] 2015	Nigeria	Nurses' general self-concept significantly mediates the relationship between job satisfaction and EE; job satisfaction and reduced PA. Nurses' general self-concept positively correlated with job satisfaction ($r = .33$; $P = .01$).
Pekcetin,[72] 2018	Turkey	Mild correlation between general satisfaction scores and PA ($r = .212$, $P < .05$); moderate negative correlation between general satisfaction scores and EE and DP ($r = -.449$, $P = .01$; $r = -.474$, $P = .01$), respectively.
Ozden et al,[65] 2013	Turkey	Correlation between job satisfaction and burnout subscale EE, DP, and PA note statistical significance ($r = -.041$, $P = .000$; $r = -.0324$, $P = .000$; $r = 0.336$, $P = .000$, respectively). Thus, nurses who suffer emotional exhaustion and depersonalization have lower scores for job satisfaction, whereas nurses who had high personal achievement experienced higher levels of job satisfaction.
Happell & Koehn,[63] 2011	Australia	No analysis of correlation between burnout and job satisfaction was reported. Nurses lacking job satisfaction would consider seclusion justifiable for inappropriate behaviors vs nurses with higher level of job satisfaction scores.
Abushaikha & Saca-Hazboun,[57] 2009	Palestine	Moderate levels of job satisfaction and burnout noted, although not significant. Most nurses reported moderate job satisfaction (84.2%) and burnout (EE 38%). Areas of low job satisfaction related to advancement (41.4%) and company policies and practices (28.9%).
Arikan et al,[19] 2007	Turkey	Nurses working in University Hospital had highest EE and lowest job satisfaction scores. Lower perceived personal success and job satisfaction scores related to the number of work hours per week (49 or more) compared with those working 40–48 h/wk. Nurses working a rotation system with night duties demonstrated lower job satisfaction scores and higher EE and DP scores.

(continued on next page)

Table 4
(continued)

Tool Used to Measure Job Satisfaction	Article Reference	Country	Findings
Job Satisfaction by Stephen Kerr	Tourigny et al,[73] 2007	Japan & China	Japanese nurses: Age positively related to job satisfaction ($r = .19$, $P < .01$). EE is positively related to DP ($r = .41$, $P < .01$) and negatively related to job satisfaction ($r = -.42$, $P < .01$). EE is negatively related to diminished PA ($r = -.17$, $P < .05$). Regression analysis results indicate DP is negatively related to job satisfaction ($r = -.31$, $P < .01$). Diminished PA is negatively related to job satisfaction ($r = -.18$, $P < .01$). Job satisfaction is a predictor of DP, diminished PA. Chinese nurses: Age is positively related to EE and job satisfaction ($R = .11$, $P < .05$; $r = 13$, $P < .01$, respectively). To DP, age negatively relates ($r = -.17$, $P < .01$) and diminished PA ($r = -.21$, $P < .01$). EE is related to DP ($r = .26$, $P < .01$). EE is negatively related to job satisfaction ($r = -.30$, $P < .01$). Diminished PA is negatively related to job satisfaction ($r = .43$, $P < .01$).
Font-Roja Questionnaire[78]	Portero de la Cruz & Vaquero Abellán,[37] 2015	Spain	No relationship noted between burnout and satisfaction. Global mean satisfaction was 66.46 ± 7.04, ranging from 51 to 85 points. MBI mean score for EE, EP, and PA were 17.48, 9.04, 39.22, respectively. A positive and significant relation was noted with professionals' age and job satisfaction (each additional year of age, job satisfaction increases by 0.22 points).
Job Satisfaction Visual Analog Scale (VAS-scale)	Vermeir et al,[14] 2018	Belgium	No significant relation with burnout. Small percentage (5.3%) of total ICU nurses (n = 300) indicated job dissatisfaction.
	Vermeir et al,[68] 2018	Belgium	No significant relation with burnout. Overall, mean job satisfaction $7.49 \pm 1.43/10$ (median = 8, IQR = 7–8.5) was high among hospital nurses. Of the 1436 nurses, 103 (7.2%) reported dissatisfaction. Dissatisfaction associated with work department, employment status (part-time), and years of experience.

Mueller-McCloskey Satisfaction Scale (MMSS)[79] Practice Environment Scale of the Nursing Work Index (PES-NWI)[26] Simplified Coping Style Questionnaire (SCSQ)[82]	Liu et al,[64] 2015	Shanghi China	Moderate correlations between burnout and job satisfaction for EE, DP, and PA (r = −0.488, −0.334, 0.328, respectively, $P < .0001$). Moderate correlations noted between job satisfaction and each practice environment subscale (nurse participation in hospital affairs, nurse foundations for quality of care, nurse manager ability, staffing/resource adequacy, nurse-physician relations; r = 0.453, 0.428, 0.431, 0.362, 0.281, respectively, $P < .0001$). Job satisfaction moderately correlated with the positive subscale of the coping style (r = 0.348, $P < .001$).
Extended Satisfaction with Life Scale[80,81]	Roulin et al,[67] 2014	Switzerland	Individual level—predictors of burnout and work-family conflict significantly predicted findings related to job satisfaction. Group level—significant predictor of job satisfaction was group cohesion and unit effectiveness. Organizational level—no magnet factors (control over practice, autonomy, and nurse-physician relationship) were significant predictors of job satisfaction.

Table 5
Recommendations to increase job satisfaction

Recommendation for	Article	Findings
Individual Nurse	Ariken et al,[19] 2007 Hayes et al,[36] 2015 Roulin et al,[67] 2014	At the individual level, a significant decrease in job satisfaction occurs when nurses experience incompatible time demand challenges between work and family.[19] Hayes et al[36] report one of the most critical factors contributing to satisfaction was flexible management and a feeling valued. To enhance nurse satisfaction and ultimately nurse retention, creating a variety of flexible work schedule options (ie, weekend-only option, buddy schedules with alternative hours, all holiday schedule, seasonal schedule) should be offered.[19,67]
Group	Khamisa et al,[35] 2016 Hayes et al,[36] 2015 Alharbi et al,[55] 2016 Liu et al,[64] 2016 Roulin et al,[67] 2014 Portero de la Cruz & Vaquero Abellán,[37] 2015	At the group level, the practice environment plays a significant role in job satisfaction; therefore, it is imperative to implement strategies fostering its improvement.[35,64] Within the work environment, taking steps necessary to improve group cohesiveness, social support system among the team, and communication between nurses and management can help improve job satisfaction.[67] Team building program is one way to foster group cohesiveness.[55] In addition, nurse managers or other nurses in a position of leadership should consider participating in staff rounds as one way to nurture and build the support system and communication processes.[68] Furthermore, to positively affect job satisfaction, encourage nurses to become involved in the processes within the unit or clinical area.[55] Lastly, routinely acknowledging nurse accomplishments and praising job performance influence feeling of success and, in turn, nurse's job satisfaction.[36,55]
Organization	Roulin et al,[67] 2014	At the organizational level, policies aimed at empowering nurses should be instituted to enhance nurses' autonomy and positively affect job satisfaction. The health care organization should grant nurses more control and freedom in making decisions regarding caring for patients.[67]

Table 6
Factors associated with workplace violence

Factors	Article	Findings
Barriers to Reporting WPV	AMN Healthcare Alameddine et al,[88] Ajoudani et al,[85] ANA,[84] International Council,[83] Merecz et al,[87]	Although 41% of nurses in a 2019 survey AMN Healthcare[88] report being a victim of WPV often, incidences are underreported due to various reasons.[83,85,87,88] Barriers to reporting can relate to one's perception and beliefs. For example, violent incidents are routine, Alameddine et al[88] considered part of the job,[88] and besides, nothing is going to be done anyways, so why waste time reporting.[84,88] Additionally, fear of retaliation or being blamed,[83] lack of proof,[83] lack of understanding or agreement about what constitutes violence,[83] and lack of training about reporting[83] and lastly, no existing WPV policies.[88]
Nurse, delivery of health care, and the organization	Alameddine et al,[88] Ajoudani et al,[85] ANA[84] International Council[83] Merecz et al[87] Lanz et al,[82]	WPV adversely affects the nurse, delivery of health care, and the organization. Depression, anxiety, stress, disturbances to sleep and appetite, as well as negatively affecting nurse victims' family and social life, are reported within the literature.[85,88] Furthermore, absenteeism, job dissatisfaction, burnout, and a lack of commitment ensues that ultimately affect both the quality of patient care and care outcomes.[85,87,88] In turn, directly and indirectly affecting the organization (ie, reputation, financial status, productivity).[82,83,85,88]
Triggers	Alameddine et al[88] Ajoudani et al[85] Lanz & Bruk-Lee,[82]	Determinants that trigger aforementioned consequences include patient (ie, mental illness; substance abuse, patient expectations)[88] and organization (ie, inadequate staffing, staff workload, waiting times, poor security)[85,88] characteristics. As well, staff variables such as age, experience, and gender[88] and interpersonal conflict. Research findings reveal younger, less experienced female nurses (<5 y' experience)[88] are more prone to verbal forms of abuse and bullying whereas younger and less experienced men (<9 y' experience)[88] were more prone to acts of physical violence. Lanz[82] research findings show a connection between interpersonal conflict and burnout; therefore, emotions are triggers that can potentially lead to WPV between employees.

Table 7
Workplace violence

Tool Used to Measure Workplace Violence	Article Reference	Country	Findings
Survey Instrument—exposure to and consequence of violence—verbal abuse and physical violence over last 12 mo	Alameddine et al,[85] 2015	Lebanon	Verbal abuse was significantly associated with burnout (EE = P < .0001; DP = P < .001; PA = P = .014). Age and years of experience variable significantly associated with verbal abuse (P = .017), as was rotation shift work (P = .039). Exposure and organization antiviolence policies and regulations showed significant link (P < .001). Moderate or high burnout related to DP and nurses subjected to physical violence significant (P = .026). Variables significantly associated were age (P = .046), gender (P = .001), nightshift work (P < .001).
Negative Acts Questionnaire Revised (NAQ-R)[89]	Ajoudani et al,[86] 2019	Iran	Correlation of burnout and bullying significant in all dimensions. Physical bullying and AE, DP, and PD (r = 0.311, 0.301, and 0.319, respectively, P < .01). Work bullying and AE, DP, and PD (r = 0.333, 0.299, and 0.342, respectively, P < .01, P < .1, P < .05). Personal bullying and AE, DP, and PD (r = 0.318, 0.403, and 0.377, respectively, P < .01). *Note—dimensions in burnout scale by authors reported burnout subscales EE, DP, and PA as AE (affective exhaustion), DP (depersonalization, and PD (personal deficit).
Stress at Work Scale[71]	Merecz et al,[87] 2006	Poland	In psychiatric nurses (PN), moderate correlation between the total aggression score and DP (rho = 0.449; P = 0.0001). The higher the level of aggression, the higher the level of EE (rho = 0.279; P = .015). In non-PN, a weak-to-moderate correlation between total aggression score and burnout. The higher the level of aggression, the higher the level of EE (rho = 0.400; P < .0001) and a stronger tendency to depersonalize patients (rho = 0.486; P < .0001), and lower PA (rho = −0.213; P = .0002).
Interpersonal Conflict at Work Scale	Lanz & Bruk-Lee,[82] 2017	United States	Interpersonal conflict at work affects burnout on each subscale EE, DP, and PA, respectively (β = .37; β = .45 β = −.37 with a significance of P < .01).

(ie, supervisors, managers, coworkers) violence does occur.[85–87] Factors associated with workplace violence are summarized in **Table 6**.

From Zangaro and colleagues'[5] systematic review, researchers hypothesized that nurse burnout might be associated with nurse workplace violence. Between the

Table 8
Workplace violence recommendations

Recommendation	Article Reference	Findings
Policies	Alameddine et al,[85] ANA[84] International Council[83]	Every health care organization should mandate antiviolence policies and specific policies governing reporting processes
Zero-Tolerance	Alameddine et al,[85] ANA[83,84] International Council[83]	A strong commitment of zero-tolerance to WPV throughout the entire industry and within each organization from the top-down is imperative to affecting positive change. In addition, due to the confusion as to what constitutes violence and faulty perceptions of acceptable behaviors about violence, heightening awareness is vital
Education Training	Alameddine et al,[85] ANA[84] International Council[83]	Educational training done annually, if not more often, should be required of all health care workers.[71,74] As well, a requisite in prelicensure programs is necessary because novice nurses are more prone to becoming victims of WPV and lack skills of managing violent situations[74]
Conflict Management	Lanz & Bruk-Lee,[82]	Reducing interpersonal conflict through training on conflict management skills can prove helpful in warding off WPV between employees

time span of 2000 to 2019, a total of 10 research studies were located within Zangaro and colleagues'[5] systematic review, of which only 4 articles retrieved met the criteria for selection (full MBI, nurses only). All articles but 1 were from outside of the United States. Instruments used to measure workplace violence and its correlation to associated factors including burnout as measured by the MBI.[4] **Table 7** presents these instruments, research article of reference, country of origin surrounding the research, and a summary of the findings.

An absence of antiviolence policies in health care settings or a lack of a straightforward, standardized process for reporting significantly affects incidents of violence.[82,86] **Table 8** summarized actions that can be taken to affect workplace violence.

In summary, WPV is a prominent and severe issue facing health care settings worldwide. WPV has detrimental consequences on those exposed to violence and the overall profession of nursing and the health care field. A system-wide cultural change and mindset toward zero-tolerance of all forms of violence can positively affect the landscape of the health care profession, the health care industry, and global society.

SUMMARY

It is apparent from the literature that nurse burnout is an ongoing problem that has potential consequences in adverse job factors and outcomes, both in the United States and internationally. In this article, research on the MBI is reviewed from 2000 to 2019, specifically analyzing job factors associated with nurse burnout and comparing US with international findings. Most of the reviewed articles found a significant relationship between nurse burnout and a nurse's intention to leave their job, job stress, nurse satisfaction, and workplace violence.

Recommendations from the reviewed articles had similar themes for interventions to lower nurse burnout in an attempt to decrease the adverse job characteristics. To lower burnout for the individual nurse, educational programs are suggested to include training in conflict management, training opportunities to increase confidence in skills, and training in ways to reduce personal stress such as meditation or mindfulness training.[34] On an organizational level efforts should be made to improve the work environment by encouraging group cohesiveness[51] with social support, improving communication between leadership and staff,[67] and team building programs.[55] Other recommendations for leadership in an organization are to find ways to reduce work-related stressors, support nurse autonomy,[51] and nurse recognition programs.[38,51] Policies should be developed to address appropriate staffing allocations,[16] increase income,[16] allow flexible work schedules,[35,64] and zero-tolerance for WPV.[82,86]

Most of the articles in systematic review were cross-sectional studies, but longitudinal studies may offer more insight into nurse burnout. More experimental type studies that look at job characteristics that are related to burnout could offer evidence to organizations to encourage leadership to provide more support to nurses.

CLINICS CARE POINTS

- Individual nurses should take opportunities to increase confidence in their skills, conflict management, and reduce personal stress.
- Organizations should take steps to create a positive work environment, by lowering stress, providing clear communication, supporting nurse autonomy, ensuring appropriate staffing allocation, providing fair income, offering flexible work schedules, and guaranteeing a zero-tolerance for WPV.

DISCLOSURE

The authors have nothing to disclose.

REFERENCES

1. World Health Organization (W.H.O.). Burn-Out an "Occupational Phenomenon": International classification of diseases. Available at: https://www.who.int/news/item/28-05-2019-burn-out-an-occupational-phenomenon-international-classification-of-diseases.
2. Freudenberger HJ. Staff burn-out. J Soc Issues 1974;30(1):159–65.
3. Maslach C, Jackson SE, Leiter MP. Maslach burnout inventory manual. 4th edition. Menlo Park (CA): Mind Garden, Inc; 2016.
4. Maslach C, Jackson SE, Schaufeli WB, et al. Maslach burnout inventory (MBI). Available at: https://www.mindgarden.com/117-maslach-burnout-inventory-mbi.
5. Zangaro GA, Dulko D, Sullivan D, et al. Systematic review of burnout in U.S. nurses. Nurs Clin North Am 57(1):29–51.
6. Williamson K, Lank PM, Cheema N, et al. Comparing the maslach burnout inventory to other well-being instruments in emergency medicine residents. J Grad Med Educ 2018;10(5):532–6.
7. Al Mutair A, Al Mutairi A, Chagla H, et al. Examining and adapting the psychometric properties of the Maslach Burnout Inventory-Health Services Survey (MBI-HSS) among Healthcare Professionals. Appl Sci 2020;10(5):1890.
8. Squires A, Finlayson C, Gerchow L, et al. Methodological considerations when translating "burnout". Burn Res 2014;1(2):59–68.

9. Loera B, Converso D, Viotti S. Evaluating the psychometric properties of the mas-lach burnout inventory-human services survey (MBI-HSS) among Italian nurses: how many factors must a researcher consider? PLoS One 2014;9(12):e114987.

10. Poghosyan L, Aiken LH, Sloane DM. Factor structure of the Maslach burnout in-ventory: an analysis of data from large scale cross-sectional surveys of nurses from eight countries. Int J Nurs Stud 2009;46(7):894–902 [Erratum appears in Int J Nurs Stud 2014;51(10):1416-1417].

11. Maslach C, Leiter MP. Understanding the burnout experience: recent research and its implications for psychiatry. World Psychiatry 2016;15(2):103–11.

12. State of the world's nursing 2020: investing in education, jobs and leadership. Geneva (Switzerland): World Health Organization; 2020.

13. Kelbach J. Improving nurse retention: six strategies to reduce RN turnover. Office of Nursing Workforce; 2020. Available at: https://www.msbn.ms.gov/onw/.

14. Vermeir P, Blot S, Degroote S, et al. Communication satisfaction and job satisfac-tion among critical care nurses and their impact on burnout and intention to leave: a questionnaire study. Intensive Crit Care Nurs 2018;48:21–7.

15. Lorenz VR, Sabino MO. Corrêa Filho HR. Professional exhaustion, quality and in-tentions among family health nurses. Rev Paul Enferm 2018;71(suppl 5): 2295–301.

16. Jiang H, Ma L, Gao C, et al. Satisfaction, burnout and intention to stay of emer-gency nurses in Shanghai. Emery Med J 2017;34(7):448–53.

17. Jourdain G, Chênevert D. Job demands–resources, burnout and intention to leave the nursing profession: a questionnaire survey. Int J Nurs Stud 2010; 47(6):709–22.

18. Leiter MP, Jackson NJ, Shaughnessy K. Contrasting burnout, turnover intention, control, value congruence and knowledge sharing between Baby Boomers and Generation X. J Nurs Manag 2009;17(1):100–9.

19. Arikan F, Koksal CD, Gokce C. Work-related stress, burnout, and job satisfaction of dialysis nurses in association with perceived relations with professional con-tacts. Dial Transplant 2007;36(4):1–191.

20. Arslan Yurumezoglu H, Kocaman G. Predictors of nurses' intentions to leave the organisation and the profession in Turkey. J Nurs Manag 2016;24(2):235–43.

21. Bruyneel L, Thoelen T, Adriaenssens J, et al. Emergency room nurses' pathway to turnover intention: a moderated serial mediation analysis. J Adv Nurs 2017;73(4): 930–42.

22. Lagerlund M, Sharp L, Lindqvist R, et al. Intention to leave the workplace among nurses working with cancer patients in acute care hospitals in Sweden. Eur J On-col Nurs 2015;19(6):629–37.

23. Meng L, Liu Y, Liu H, et al. Relationships among structural empowerment, psy-chological empowerment, intent to stay and burnout in nursing field in mainland China—based on a cross-sectional questionnaire research. Int J Nurs Pract 2015;21(3):303–12.

24. Pienaar JW, Bester CL. The impact of burnout on the intention to quit among pro-fessional nurses in the Free State region—A national crisis? South Afr J Psy 2011; 41(1):113–22.

25. van Veldhoven M, Meijman TF. Measuring psychosocial workload with a question-naire: the questionnaire experience and assessment of work (VBBA). Amsterdam NIA 1994.

26. Lake ET. Development of the practice environment scale of the Nursing Work In-dex. Res Nurs Health 2002;25(3):176–88. https://doi.org/10.1002/nur.10032.

27. Van der Doef M, Maes S. (1999) The job demand-control (-Support) model and psychological well-being: a review of 20 years of empirical research. Work Stress 2015;13:87–114.
28. Kim S, Price JL, Mueller CW, et al. The determinants of career intent among physicians at a U.S. Air Force Hospital. Hum Relat 1996;49:947–76.
29. Maslach C, Leiter M. Understanding the burnout experience: Recent research and its implications for psychiatry. World Psychiatry 2016;15(2):103–11.
30. Liao RW, Yeh ML, Lin KC, et al. A Hierarchical model of occupational burnout in nurses associated with job-induced stress, self-concept, and work environment. J Nurs Res 2020;28(2):e79.
31. World Health Organization. Occupational health:Stress at the workplace. 19 October 2020. Available at: https://www.who.int/news-room/q-a-detail/ccupational-health-stress-at-the-workplace.
32. Veda A, Roy R. Occupational stress among nurses: a forctrial study with special reference to Indore City. J Health Manag 2020;22(1):67–77.
33. Luan X, Wang P, Hou W, et al. Job stress and burnout: a comparative study of senior and head nurses in China. Nurs Health Sci 2017;19(2):163–9.
34. Liao R-W, Yeh M-L, Lin K-C, et al. A Hierarchical model of occupational burnout in nurses associated with job-induced stress, self-concept, and work environment. J Nurs Res 2020;28(2):e79.
35. Khamisa N, Peltzer K, Ilic D, et al. Work related stress, burnout, job satisfaction and general health of nurses: a follow-up study. Int J Nurs Pract 2016;22(6):538–45.
36. Hayes B, Bonner A, Douglas C. Haemodialysis work environment contributors to job satisfaction and stress: a sequential mixed methods study. BMC Nurs 2015;14:58.
37. Portero de la Cruz S, Vaquero Abellán M. Professional burnout, stress and job satisfaction of nursing staff at a university hospital. Rev Lat Am Enfermagem 2015;23(3):543–52.
38. Adriaenssens J, De Gucht V, Maes S. Causes and consequences of occupational stress in emergency nurses, a longitudinal study. J Nurs Manag 2015;23(3):346–58.
39. McTiernan K, McDonald N. Occupational stressors, burnout and coping strategies between hospital and community psychiatric nurses in a Dublin region. J Psychiatr Ment Health Nurs 2015;22(3):208–18.
40. Tuna R, Baykal Ü. The relationship between job stress and burnout levels of oncology nurses. Asia Pac J Oncol Nurs 2014;1(1):33–9.
41. Jaracz M, Rosiak I, Bertrand-Bucińska A, et al. Affective temperament, job stress and professional burnout in nurses and civil servants. PLoS One 2017;12(6). https://doi.org/10.1371/journal.pone.0176698.
42. Jamal M, Baba VV. Job stress and burnout among Canadian managers and nurses: an empirical examiniation. Can J Public Health 2000;91(6):454–8.
43. Assadi T, Sadeghi F, Noyani A, et al. Occupational burnout and its related factors among Iranian nurses: A cross-sectional study in shahroud, northeast of Iran. Open Access Maced J Med Sci 2019;7(17):2902–7.
44. Li XM, Liu YJ. Job stressors and burnout among staff nurses. Chin J Nurs 2000;35:645–9 (in Chinese).
45. Benoliel JQ, McCorkle R, Georgiadou F, et al. Measurement of stress in clinical nursing. Cancer Nurs 1990;13(4):221–8.
46. Rothmann S, Van Der Colff JJ, Rothmann JC. Occupational stress of nurses in South Africa. Curationis 2006;29:24–5.

47. Escribà V, Más R, Cárdenas M, et al. Validación de la escala de estresores laborales en personal de enfermería: "the nursing stress scale". Gac Sanit 1999;13(3): 191–200.

48. Gelsema T, van der Doef M, Maes S, et al. Job stress in the nursing profession: the influence of organizational and environmental conditions and job characteristics. Int J Stress Manag 2005;12(3):222–40.

49. Cushway D, Tyler A, Nolan P. Development of a stress scale for mental health professionals. Br J Clin Psychol 1996;35:279–95.

50. Güngör, S. Türk örnekleminde is stresi ve sosyal desteðin tükenmislik üzerindeki etkileri (effects of job stressors and social support on burnout in a Turkish sample). Boðaziçi Üniversitesi Sosyal Bilimler Enstitüsü, Yükseklisans Tezi (Bogazici University Institute of Social Sciences, Unpublished Master Thesis). 1997.

51. Revicki DA, May HJ, Whitley TW. Reliability and validity of the Work-Related Strain Inventory among health professionals. Behav Med Fall 1991;17(3):111–20.

52. Hayes G, Bonner A, Pryor J. Factors contributing to nurse job satisfaction in the acute care hospital setting: a review of recent literature. J Nurs Manag 2010; 18(7):804–14.

53. Payne A, Koen L, Niehaus DJH, et al. Burnout and job satisfaction of nursing staff in South African acute mental health setting. S Afri J Psychiat 2020;26(0):1454.

54. Aiken LH, Sermeus W, Van Den Heede K, et al. Patient safety, satisfaction, and quality of hospital care: cross sectional surveys of nurses and patients in 12 countries in Europe and the United States. BMJ 2012;344(7851):1–14.

55. Alharbi J, Wilson R, Woods C, et al. The factors influencing burnout and job satisfaction among critical care nurses: a study of Saudi critical care nurses. J Nurs Manag 2016;24(7):708–17.

56. Adwan JZ. Pediatric nurses' grief experience, burnout and job satisfaction. J Pediatr Nurs 2014;29(4):329–36.

57. Abushaikha L, Saca-Hazboun H. Job satisfaction and burnout among Palestinian nurses. East Mediterr Health J 2009;15(1):190–7. Available at: http://www.emro. who.int/emhj-volume-15-2009/volume-15-issue-1/Page-1.html.

58. Hayes B, Douglas C, Bonner A. Work environment, job satisfaction, stress and burnout among haemodialysis nurses. J Nurs Manag 2015;23(5):588–98.

59. Nwafor CE, Immanel EU, Obi-Nwosu H. Does nurses'self-concept mediate the relationship between job satisfaction and burnout among Nigerian nurses. Int J Afr Nurs Sci 2015;3:71–5.

60. Utriainen K, Kyngas H. Hospital nurses' job satisfaction: a literature review. J Nurs Manag 2009;17(8):1002–10.

61. Van der Doef M, Mbazzi FB, Verhoeven C. Job conditions, job satisfaction, somatic complaints and burnout among East African nurses. J Clin Nurs 2012; 21(11–12):1763–75.

62. Zangara GA, Soeken KL. A meta-analysis of studies of nurses' job satisfaction. Res Nurs Health 2007;30(4):445–58.

63. Happell B, Koehn S. Seclusion as a necessary intervention: the relationship between burnout, job satisfaction and therapeutic optimism and justification for the use of seclusion. J Adv Nurs 2011;67(6):1222–31.

64. Liu YE, While A, Li SJ, et al. Job satisfaction and work related variables in Chinese cardiac critical care nurses. J Nurs Manag 2015;23(5):487–97.

65. Ozden D, Karagozoglu S, Yildirim G. Intensive care nurses' perception of futility: Job satisfaction and burnout dimensions. Nurs Ethics 2013;20(4):436–47.

66. Palazoglu CA, Koc Z. Ethical sensitivity, burnout, and job satisfaction in emergency nurses. Nurs Ethics 2019;26(3):809–22.

67. Roulin N, Mayor E, Bangerter A. How to satisfy and retain personnel despite job-market shortage: multilevel predictors of nurses' job satisfaction and intent to leave. Swiss J Psychol 2014;73(1):13–24.

68. Vermeir P, Downs C, Degroote S, et al. Intraorganizational communication and job satisfaction among Flemish hospital nurses: an exploratory multicenter study. Workplace Health Saf 2018;66(1):16–23.

69. Akman O, Ozturk C, Bektas M, et al. Job satisfaction and burnout among paediatric nurses. J Nurs Manag 2016;24(7):923–33.

70. Pinikahana J, Happell B. Stress, burnout and job satisfaction in rural psychiatric nurses: a Victorian study. Aust J Rural Health 2004;12(3):120–5.

71. Topbas E, Bay H, Turan BB, et al. The effect of perceived organisational justice on job satisfaction and burnout levels of haemodialysis nurses. J Ren Care 2019; 45(2):120–8.

72. Pekcetin S. Ageist attitudes and their association with burnout and job satisfaction among nursing staff: a descriptive study. Turk Geriatri Derg 2018;21(1): 25–32.

73. Tourigny L, Baba VV, Wang X. Burnout and depression among nurses in Japan and China: the moderating effects of job satisfaction and absence. Int J Hum Resour Manag 2010;21(15):2741–61.

74. van der Doef M, Maes S. The Leiden Quality of Work Questionnaire: its construction, factor structure, and psychometric qualities. Psychol Rep 1999;85(3 Pt 1): 954–62. https://doi.org/10.2466/pr0.1999.85.3.954.

75. Stamps P. Nurses and work satisfaction: an index for measurement. Chicago (IL): Health Administration Press; 1997.

76. Spector PE. Job satisfaction: application, assessment, causes, and consequences. Thousand. Oaks (CA): Sage; 1997.

77. Weiss DJ, Davis RV, England GW, et al. Manual for the Minnesota satisfaction questionnaire: occupational psychology research. Minneapolis: University of Minnesota; 1967. p. 1–119.

78. Aranaz J, Mira J. Cuestionario Font Roja. Un instrument de medida de la satisfaccion en el medio hospitalario. Todo Hosp 1988;52:63–6.

79. Mueller CP, McCloskey JC. Nurses' job satisfaction: a proposed measure. Nurs Res 1990;39(2):113–7.

80. Jie YN. Simplified coping style questionnaire: reliability and validity assessment. Chin J Clin Psychol 1998;2:53–4.

81. Alfonso VC, Allison DB, Rader DE, et al. The extended satisfaction with life scale: development and psychometric properties. Soc Indic Res 1996;38:275–301.

82. Lanz JJ, Bruk-Lee V. Resilience as a moderator of the indirect effects of conflict and workload on job outcomes among nurses. J Adv Nurs 2017;73:2973–86.

83. International Council of Nurses. Position statement. Prevention and management of workplace violence. Available at: https://www.icn.ch/sites/default/files/inline-files/PS_C_Prevention_mgmt_workplace _violence.pdf.

84. American Nurses Association. Reporting incidents of workplace violence. Available at: https://www.nursingworld.org/globalassets/practiceandpolicy/work-environment/endnurseabuse/endabuse-issue-brief-final.pdf.

85. Alameddine M, Mourad Y, Dimassi H. A national study on nurses' exposure to occupational violence in Lebanon: prevalence, consequences and associated factors. PLoS One 2015;10(9):1–15.

86. Ajoudani F, Baghaei R, Lotfi M. Moral distress and burnout in Iranian nurses: the mediating effect of workplace bullying. Nurs Ethics 2019;26(6):1834–47.

87. Merecz D, Rymaszewska J, Moscicka A, et al. Violence at the workplace – a questionnaire survey of nurses. Eur Psychiatry 2006;21(7):442–50.
88. AMN Healthcare. 2019 Survey registered nurses a challenging decade ahead. Available at: https://www.amnhealthcare.com/2019-survey-of-registered-nurses-a-challenging-decade-ahead/.
89. Nowicka M, Kolasa W. [Being faced with an aggressive client—psychological consequences for employees] W obliczu agresywnego petenta— konsekwencje psychologiczne dla pracowników. Med Pr 2001;1:1–5.

Comparison of Factors Associated with Physician and Nurse Burnout

Dorothy Dulko, PhD, ARNP-BC, AOCNP, WHNP-BC[1],*,
George A. Zangaro, PhD, RN, FAAN[1]

KEYWORDS

- Burnout • Nurse • Physician • Maslach • Coping strategies • Mindfulness

KEY POINTS

- The World Health Organization (WHO) has acknowledged the serious consequences of physician and nurse burnout.
- Recent research revealed that nearly 80% of registered nurses and more than 50% of physicians reported experiencing burnout.
- Coping strategies such as mindfulness seem to mitigate the effects of burnout in both nurses and physicians and should be fostered at the individual and organizational level.

INTRODUCTION

Burnout syndrome has been defined by Maslach as a state of chronic stress characterized by high levels of emotional exhaustion (EE) and depersonalization (DP) and low levels of professional effectiveness.[1] The Maslach Burnout Inventory Human Services Survey (MBI- HSS) is a widely used self-administered survey widely used to assess burnout among health care providers. The MBI- HSS uses 22 items to assess levels of 3 dimensions: (1) EE (9 items), (2) DP (5 items), and (3) feelings of personal accomplishment (PA) (8 items). Each item is scored using a 7-level scale ranging from 0 to 6 (from never to every day), allowing for subscale assessment in all 3 dimensions.[2]

The World Health Organization (WHO) has acknowledged the serious consequences of health care worker burnout resulting from persistent workplace stress, reporting burnout levels among physicians and nurses at new highs and consistently increasing.[3] A recent study revealed that nearly 80% of registered nurses (RN)

American Association of Colleges of Nursing (AACN), 655 K Street NW, Suite 750, Washington, DC 20001, USA
[1] The views, analyses, and conclusions expressed in this article are those of the authors and do not necessarily reflect the official policy or positions of the American Association of Colleges of Nursing.
* Corresponding author.
E-mail address: dorothydulko@gmail.com

reported experiencing burnout.[4] In 2017, the National Academy of Medicine (NAM) action collaborative on clinician well-being and resilience began exploring ways to enhance the understanding of clinician well-being, raise the visibility of clinician stress and burnout, and promote evidenced-based, multidisciplinary solutions.[5]

BACKGROUND- BURNOUT

Included in the 11th Revision of the International Classification of Diseases (ICD-11), burnout is a condition resulting from chronic workplace stress that has not been effectively managed, described within 3 dimensions: (a) feelings of energy depletion or exhaustion, (b) increased mental distance from one's job, and (c) reduced professional efficacy.[3] Burnout is a widespread phenomenon in health care reaching concerning levels among United States (US) health care professionals, with some studies reporting more than 50% of physicians and one-third of nurses reporting symptoms.[6] Burnout is especially prevalent among physicians in training.

The growing incidence of reported burnout has been identified as a possible risk to patient safety, with physicians who experience signs of burnout expressing concern about making medical errors.[7] High levels of nurse burnout have been associated with poor patient perception of care quality,[8] higher patient mortality, and an increase in health care-associated infections.[6] Nurses and physicians who suffer with symptoms of burnout may experience problems outside of the workplace including substance abuse, suicidal ideation, and difficulty with interpersonal relationships.[9] Having less than 5 years of work experience and more working hours per week are among the factors that seem to increase the risk for health care provider burnout.[10]

Addressing health care provider burnout, specifically as experienced by physicians and nurses, is a priority health care policy goal.[11] Identifying risk factors and devoting resources to improving physicians' and nurses' welfare are now viewed as vital to meeting health care organization aims.[12] It is imperative to evaluate the factors associated with physician and nurse burnout and to develop strategies that address the individual and organizational factors that contribute to this health care priority.

Factors Associated with Physician and Nurse Burnout - A Scoping Review

Methods

To determine the factors associated with burnout in nurses and physicians, a scoping review was conducted to identify key variables that are related to burnout in these health care professionals. A systematic search process was conducted following the preferred reporting items for systematic reviews and meta-analysis (PRISMA) guidelines[13] .

A librarian performed a systematic search using the following databases: PubMed, CINAHL, Medline, PsycInfo, ProQuest, Embase, Cochrane, ERIC, and TRIP. The databases were searched from January 2000 to December 2019. The search terms included: "burnout," "burn-out," "burn out," "Maslach," and "nurse." A Boolean strategy using the operators AND and OR enhanced the searches and ensured a comprehensive search was completed.

Inclusion criteria

Studies were included in the review if they met the following criteria: (a) the study was a quantitative analysis of empirical data using the MBI- HSS, (b) all 3 subscales of the 22-item MBI were used, (c) the sample consisted of RN and/or physicians, (d) sample size for the study was reported, (e) variables reported in the study had a significant correlation from univariate, multivariate, and logistic regression analyses with any of the MBI subscales, (f) the study was published between 2000 and 2019, (g) study setting was in the United States, and (h) the study was published in English. Studies before 2000 were not included because care delivery approaches were evolving, with improvements in the efficiency of care being adopted. Studies conducted outside of the United States were excluded because the health care systems and practice environments differ in counties outside of the United States when compared with U.S. health care organizations.

Study screening process

Fig. 1 provides a summary of the systematic search process. The search of electronic databases yielded 6533 titles and abstracts. After the removal of duplicates, non-English articles, and conference abstracts or presentations, there were 2391 titles and abstracts screened for inclusion. The titles and abstracts of articles were independently screened by 2 members of the research team to determine if the inclusion criteria were met. Any disagreements were discussed until consensus was reached. Articles were excluded if both reviewers agreed that the inclusion criteria were not met. Five hundred and twelve nursing articles and 415 physician articles were screened for eligibility. Following the completion of screening, 16 nursing studies and 22 physician studies met the inclusion criteria and were included in the scoping review. The most common reasons for the exclusion of studies from the review were: (a) studies did not use all 22-items on the MBI-HSS, (b) studies did not report correlations, and (c) studies were not conducted in the United States. There were 284 studies that did not use the complete version of the MBI- HSS. The majority of

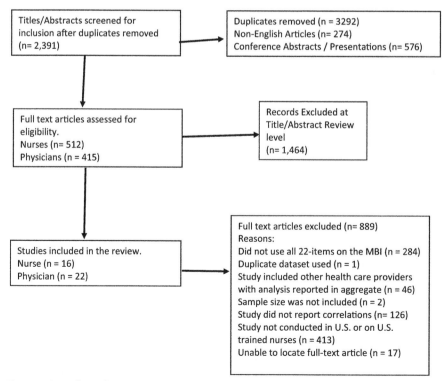

Fig. 1. Prisma flow diagram.

these studies only used the EE subscale or a combination of the EE with the DP or PA subscales. According to guidance from Maslach and colleagues,[14] using 1 or 2 of the subscales is not adequate to measure burnout. They recommend that all 3 subscales should be used to ensure adequate representation of the construct of burnout, to maintain consistency, and to allow comparability with prior research findings. Therefore, only studies using all 3 subscales were included in this review. **Table 1** presents the details of the included studies.

Data abstraction
The following data were extracted from each of the studies:

- Authors,
- year of publication,
- specialty area and,
- variables correlating with burnout. **Table 2** outlines the factors that were correlated with burnout in the studies included in this review.

Data abstraction was conducted by 2 independent reviewers and all disagreements were resolved by consensus.

Summary of the Evidence

In this scoping review, workload, work environment, satisfaction, coping mechanisms, and demographics were similar in both nurses and physicians. Physician studies more frequently reported correlations with work–life balance, patient care concerns, and health and well-being with burnout.

Demographic variables
Demographic variables such as age, gender, years of experience, and degree levels were associated with both physician and nurse burnout.[15–24] In physician studies, gender was associated with burnout revealing that women have increased odds of higher levels of burnout when compared with men.[15,16] Hyman[17] found the opposite with regard to gender, reporting that men reported a greater risk of burnout in the DP and PA scales as compared with women. Regarding EE, women reported higher EE scores as compared with men. In 2 studies, physicians over 40 years old reported higher EE scores as compared with physicians less than age 40.[17,19]

There were several demographic factors associated with nurse burnout. The older a nurse becomes, the less likely he or she is to experience higher levels of EE and DP conversely, these nurses are more likely to report increased levels of PA[10,23,24]. Similarly, nurses with more years of experience reported decreased levels of EE and DP and increased levels of PA.[22,25] In contrast, Davis[21] reported that younger nurses had significantly less levels of EE as compared with nurses older than 40 years of age. Card[20] reported that male nurses were more likely to experience higher DP scores and females reported higher EE scores. Diploma nurses reported significantly higher EE scores as compared with bachelor's prepared nurses.[20]

Workload
Workload is a major concern for both nurses and physicians, evidenced by research supporting that as workload increased, burnout increased, for example, the EE and DP subscale scores on the MBI-HSS both increased, and the PA scale score decreased. Physician studies evaluated workload using self-report measures such as number of hours worked, total hours on call and, number of weekend days worked each week.[15,19,26–28] Higher levels of burnout were consistently associated with

| Table 1 |
| Studies included in scoping review |

Physician Studies

Study Author (Year)	Specialties	Factors Associated with Burnout
Attenello et al,[35] 2018	Neurosurgery residents	Exercise, inadequate operating room exposure, poor control over schedules, social stressors outside of work, underappreciated by patients or staff
Bundy et al,[15] 2019	Interventional radiologists	Gender, workload
Campbell et al,[16] 2010	Internal medicine residents	Depression, gender
Doolittle et al,[53] 2013	Internal medicine residents	Emotional coping, spirituality
Dyrbye et al,[26] 2013	Multiple	Career satisfaction, intent to leave, work–life balance, workload
Eckleberry-Hunt et al,[48] 2017	Family physicians	Mental health status, workload
Eckleberry-Hunt et al,[33] 2009	Multiple	Alcohol and drugs, pessimism, wellness factors
Evans and Ghosh[37] 2015	Multiple	Career satisfaction, work–life balance
Fargen et al,[36] 2019	Neurointerventionalists	Feeling unappreciated by leadership, workload
Govardhan et al,[44] 2012	Multiple	Depression
Hyman et al,[17] 2009	Anesthesiologists	Age, gender, mental health, personal and professional support
Krasner et al,[49] 2009	Multiple	Mindfulness
Lu et al,[40] 2015	Emergency physicians	Career satisfaction, depression, suboptimal patient care practices
Marchalik et al,[27] 2019	Urology residents	Lack of formal mentorship, lack of mental health services, workload
Ramey et al,[28] 2017	Radiation oncology residents	Work–life balance, workload
Shanafelt et al,[38] 2002	Internal medicine residents	Suboptimal patient care practices, work–life balance, workload
Shenoi et al,[45] 2018	Pediatric physicians	Career satisfaction, exercise, gender, intent to leave, mental health, psychological distress
Simons et al,[46] 2016	Orthopedic residents and staff physicians	Career satisfaction
Streu et al,[19] 2014	Plastic Surgeons	Age, workload
West et al,[41] 2009	Internal medicine residents	Medical errors
West et al,[42] 2006	Internal medicine residents	Self-perceived medical errors

(*continued on next page*)

Table 1
(continued)

Physician Studies		
Williamson et al,[39] 2018	Emergency medicine residents	Career satisfaction, depression screening, work–life balance

Nurse Studies		
Study Author (Year)	**Specialties**	**Factors Associated with Burnout**
Adwan JZ[43] 2014	Pediatric nurses	Grief, job satisfaction
Browning et al,[52] 2006	Multiple	Cognitive adaptation, control
Card et al,[20] 2019	PeriAnesthesia nurses	Age, control, mindfulness, physical and mental health, professional support, work satisfaction
Clubbs et al 2019	Neonatal Intensive Care nurses	Developmental Care Partner Program
Davis et al,[21] 2013	Oncology nurses	Age, job satisfaction, relationship with coworkers, spirituality
Gallagher R and Gormley, DK[22] 2009	Bone marrow transplant nurses	Support systems, work schedules, years as a nurse
Gueritault-Chalvin et al,[23] 2000	Multiple	Age, control, external coping strategies, workload
Jameson BE & Bowen F[32], 2020	School nurses	Control, work environment, workload
Lanz JJ & Bruk-Lee V[30] 2017	Multiple	Interpersonal conflict, turnover, workload
Mealer et al,[50] 2012	Intensive Care Unit nurses	Resilience
Meltzer LS & Huckabay, LM[24] 2004	Critical care nurses	Age, moral distress, spirituality
Messmer et al,[47] 2004	Pediatric nurses	Work satisfaction
Muir KJ & Keim-Malpass J[31] 2019	Emergency Room nurses	Mindfulness, work environment, workload
Peery AI[29] 2010	Multiple	Caring and connecting with patients, supportive work environment, workload
Rainbow JG & Steege LM[34] 2019	Multiple	Presenteeism, stress, work environment
Russell K,[25] 2016	Oncology nurses	Lack of resources, collaboration, work environment, workload, years as a nurse

Table 2 Factors associated with burnout			
Factors Associated with Burnout	**Conceptual Definition**	**Number of Studies**	
		RN	MD
Workload	Work related duties to include work schedules, patient load, work demands, resources	8	9
Work Environment	Relationships with peers and patients, personal and professional support, mentorship	7	4
Work–life Balance	Achieving a balance between work and personal life	0	6
Patient Care Concerns	Providing suboptimal care, grief, errors	1	4
Satisfaction	Career satisfaction, job/work satisfaction, intent to leave	5	7
Health and well-being	Depression screening, drug use, overall physical and mental health	1	10
Coping mechanisms	Spirituality, cognitive adaptation, psychological factors such as mindfulness and resilience	8	2
Demographics	Age, gender, years of experience, degree levels	6	4

increased work hours. Nursing studies evaluated workload using self-report measures such as patient acuity, number of patients assigned per shift, number of hours worked each week, and amount of overtime beyond scheduled hours was worked.[23,29–33] Across all studies, workload was associated with increased burnout in nurses specifically, increased EE.

Work–life balance

A healthy work environment including the balance between the physical, intellectual, and spiritual experiences, coupled with staff empowerment, was associated with lower levels of burnout and turnover in both nurses and physicians.[17,21,25–27,29–36] In a multivariate analysis, Attenello[36] found that higher levels of burnout were reported by physicians who felt unappreciated by patients or staff, experienced hostile coresidents or faculty and experienced coresident attrition. Physicians who perceived personal and professional support with appreciation from leadership had lower EE scores and were less likely to leave the profession.[17,26,36] In a study of urology residents, a lack of formal mentorship was associated with increased burnout.[27] Support from coworkers and reduced interpersonal conflict were factors associated with lower levels of burnout and nurses' intent to leave their position.[21,30] When a nurse has a greater connection with the patient and family, EE and DP scores decrease while PA increases, resulting in a decline in reported burnout.[25,29] A study of school nurses found that a satisfactory, supportive work environment was related to little or no burnout.[32] Early career nurses with less than 1 year of practice and second-career nurses seem to experience increased rates of stress, burnout and lost productivity, all associated with a poor work environment.[34] Studies that measured work–life balance were more prominent in the medicine literature with physicians who perceived a positive work–life balance reporting lower levels of burnout.[26,37–39] Across these studies, high rates of EE were associated with perceived unsatisfactory work–life balance.

Patient safety

Patient care concerns were discussed in 4 of the physician studies. Two of these studies presented physicians reporting the feeling that they were providing suboptimal patient care, measured using self-reported patient care experiences.[39,40] In both studies, the physicians who reported higher levels of burnout also reported perceiving that they were increasingly performing suboptimal patient care practices. Two additional physician studies reported an association between an increase in medical errors and higher reported burnout.[41,42] In both of these studies, medical errors were self-reported by physicians. One nursing study described increased levels of grief in pediatric nurses who experienced the death of a patient related to increased burnout, specifically EE.[43]

Satisfaction with career and turnover

Physicians and nurses who are satisfied with their career, job, and work consistently reported an inverse association with burnout.[20,21,26,30,38–40,43–47] Among the physician studies, burnout was associated with lower career satisfaction and intent to stay in the profession.[26,38–40,45,46] One study of military physicians that indicated high overall burnout was associated with not choosing the same specialty (orthopedics) again related to lack of career satisfaction. These findings are consistent with other studies conducted in civilian facilities.[46] Early career physicians as well as residents experienced an increased level of EE and DP when compared with middle and late-career physicians.[26,40,46] Using a univariate or a multivariate model, job satisfaction of nurses was inversely correlated with EE and intent to leave the health care organization.[20,21,30,43] EE and turnover intentions typically explain the largest percent of variance in burnout. Nurses who recommended nursing as a career to others, without any reservations, had higher job satisfaction and experienced less burnout as compared with nurses who expressed reservations in recommended nursing as a career.[47]

Health and wellbeing

The concept of health and well-being was prominent in the physician studies.[16,17,27,33,39,40,44,45,48] Physical exercise was associated with decreased burnout.[35,45] Depression and mental health status were found to be positively associated with burnout and to predict burnout in multivariate modeling.[16,17,39,40,44,45,48] Unavailable or difficult to access mental health services was associated with more reported burnout in physicians.[27] Increased use of alcohol was associated with higher EE and higher DP scores in physicians.[33] In the same study, the use of prescription drugs was associated with decreased burnout in these physicians.[33]

Health and well-being of nurses were measured using self-report scales with analyses revealing that nurses who reported burnout had associated poorer physical and mental health, lower job satisfaction, believed they were less supported, perceived less opportunity for advancement, and felt that they had less control over their workload. Increased alcohol consumption and use of prescribed pain relievers was correlated with increased levels of burnout in nurses.[20]

Coping mechanisms

Several different types of coping mechanisms were reported in the literature. Mindfulness-based interventions were associated with decreased burnout in primary care physicians.[49] Two nursing studies investigated the psychological factor of mindfulness and its relationship to burnout,[20,31] with Card[20] reporting that nurses who engaged in creative or mindfulness activities, such as art, music, yoga, meditation, and prayer, experienced a significant decrease in the level of burnout. Muir[31] provided mindfulness education to nurses and reported a resultant significant reduction in burnout levels following the mindfulness educational intervention. Qualitative interviews confirmed the positive impact of mindfulness education on nurses' resiliency and identified opportunities to address burnout from a holistic perspective. Higher levels of resilience in nursing staff associated with the absence of burnout, posttraumatic stress, depression, and anxiety.[50]

A Developmental Care Partner Program was initiated in a neonatal intensive care unit at a community hospital.[51] In this program, volunteers were assigned a neonate to whom they provided sensory stimulation and appropriate developmental supportive care. The volunteers did not provide any medical care beyond the sensory exposure. Following the implementation of this program nurse burnout, specifically EE and DP were significantly reduced.

The effects of cognitive adaptation, including mastery, optimism, and self-esteem, were evaluated for their effect on work-related expectations and burnout.[52] In a large sample of nurses from multiple specialty areas, cognitive adaptation predicted fewer unmet expectations of control, which resulted in decreased reported nurse burnout. Cognitive adaptation, as well as optimism and self-esteem, were associated with a significant decrease in EE and DP scores with an increase in PA. Nurses who have an internal locus of control report feeling that they can influence their environment, while those who have an external locus of control tend to believe events as being luck or chance related to factors external to themselves. Gueritault-Chalvin[23] used a self-report instrument to measure nurses' internal and external perception of control to determine if they applied internal or external influence when attributing causality to events. Both internal and external coping strategies were reported to predict burnout, for example, nurses who use internal coping strategies feel they are in control of their environment and report lower burnout levels. External coping strategies were associated with higher levels of burnout in nursing staff.

Spirituality was identified as a coping strategy used by nurses to prevent or reduce EE.[21,24] Nurses who had no religion in their lives had significantly higher EE scores as compared with nurses who reported having religion in their lives. The use of spirituality at some level was especially important in reducing stress when nurses were faced with an ethical dilemma. Spirituality is inversely associated with EE and DP scores and positively associated with PA in physicians.[53]

SUMMARY AND DISCUSSION

Burnout is a widespread phenomenon that has reached alarming levels among United States (US) physicians and nurses with research increasingly associating burnout with more medical errors, negative impact on patient satisfaction, and quality of care. Health care provider burnout is a priority that must be addressed at the individual and organizational levels. Physician and nurse dissatisfaction has been correlated with burnout, with lower reported burnout associated with greater professional satisfaction.

The reported relationship between workload, work environment, satisfaction, coping mechanisms, demographics, and burnout are similar in nurses and physicians. Feeling empowered by a perceived healthy work–life balance, including intellectual and spiritual experiences, has been associated with lower levels of burnout in both physicians and nurses. Hostile coworkers, lack of professional support from organizational leadership, and lack of mentorship have been specifically related to higher reported physician burnout and attrition. Interpersonal conflict and lack of coworker cooperation negatively impact nurse burnout and intent to leave their position. Early career physicians and nurses both seem to be at higher risk of EE and DP when compared with their middle and late-career colleagues. The fiscal implications of health care provider burnout to organizations are clear. It has been reported that more than $4 billion in costs can be related to physician turnover and reduced clinical hours each year.[54] The cost of a nurse leaving their position is estimated to be from $11,000 to $90,000 per nurse with up to $8.5 million in associated organizational costs, including training and orientation.[55]

The aging of the nurse workforce represents an imperative to nurse retention. In 2020, the median age of RN was 52 years, up from 51 years in 2017.[56] With an increasingly older nursing workforce and early career nurses at particular risk for burnout and attrition, special care must be provided to foster retention as novice nurses transition from student to practicing nurse. Evidence suggests that physicians in training are also a particularly high-risk group for burnout due to excessive work demands, and poor work–life balance with postgraduate training requirements conflicting with personal life, affecting physician trainee work–life balance. Satisfying work relationships and collegial support seem to mitigate the effects of burnout in nurses and physicians supporting the importance of further research and integration of Team Science as a collaborative effort to address a scientific challenge, leveraging the strengths and expertise of professionals trained in different fields.

Medical errors and poor patient satisfaction related to provider burnout have been reported in both the nursing and medical literature. With patient safety and satisfaction foundational to the provision of quality health care, organizations are increasingly aware of the need to address and implement measures to foster a healthy workplace environment. The National Academy of Medicine (NAM) collaboration, including more than 200 organizations, has committed to reversing trends of increasing clinician burnout and has acknowledged the seriousness of burnout and resultant impact on patient safety, quality of care, and cost. The NAM collaborative defines burnout using the MBI subscales of EE, DP, and PA. The variables identified in this review are consistent with the consequences of burnout described by the NAM collaborative. In support of clinician well-being and improving communication between clinicians, patients, and the interdisciplinary team, NAM acknowledges the importance of an engaged workforce and visibility of clinician burnout. The NAM collaboration has committed to investing in research and information distribution to promote evidence-based solutions at the individual and system levels. The collaborative has been extended until 2022 to allow additional time to identify evidenced-based strategies to decrease provider burnout and improve clinician well-being.

Coping mechanisms represent a promising approach to reducing burnout in both nurses and physicians. Mindfulness and development of resilience strategies have been identified as key influences in reducing burnout turnover; both deserve further study. Early career turnover is a concern for individual nurses and health care organizations. Work–life balance when incorporated with supportive leadership behaviors empowers nursing staff and can be helpful in reducing burnout. Empowering leadership behaviors, including ensuring that staff are able to access the resources and support needed to perform their work, is vital. Spirituality has been shown to be a protective factor to developing burnout in health care providers. Individual and organizational interventions that targeted individual internal coping strategies, including spirituality, should be emphasized and encouraged specifically fostering those strategies that the individual he or she has identified.

Future Directions

Lack of organizational support and perception of poor practice environments contribute to physician and nurse burnout. Adequate resources, autonomy, and respectful, supportive relationships with colleagues seem to be alleviating factors. While research has largely focused on nurse and physician burnout, there is less research that specifically evaluates burnout in advanced practice providers (APPs), for example, nurse practitioners (NPs) and physician assistants. While this review has identified key factors and consequences associated with physician and nurse burnout, it is difficult to know how this applies to APPs. Bearing in mind that NPs are often trained by medical colleagues yet practice within the professional discipline of nursing, specifically studying the effect of NP role identity on burnout is warranted.

The stress and resultant burnout experienced by nurses and physicians during the COVID-19 pandemic has yet to be adequately studied or understood. While the well-being and mental health of essential workers such as physicians and nurses has been highlighted during the pandemic, evaluating the optimal mix of work–life balance and impact on burnout, studied across different timepoints, may offer deeper insight into the individual and organizational protective factors. The experience of compassion satisfaction felt by those nurses and physicians perceiving the value of team and contributing to the greater societal good deserve further study postpandemic.

Historically, employers and employees did not routinely discuss personal issues at the workplace. With clear evidence of the interwoven relationship of professional and personal life, what have been "hands-off" topics regarding personal stress must have a place of open communication within health care organizations. It is impossible to completely separate personal and professional experiences, expecting employees and colleagues to thrive personally when they are struggling professionally and vice versa. A holistic approach to health care provider well-being demands attention to the needs of the entire person-nurse or physician, with emphasis on the integral relationship between the 2.

DISCLOSURE

The authors have nothing to disclose.

REFERENCES

1. Maslach C, Schaufeli WB, Leiter MP. Job burnout. Annu Rev Psychol 2001;52: 397–422.

2. Trockel M, Bohman B, Lesure E, et al. A brief instrument to assess both burnout and professional fulfillment in physicians: reliability and validity, including correlation with self-reported medical errors, in a sample of resident and practicing physicians. Acad Psychiatry 2018;42(1):11–24.

3. World Health Organization (WHO). Burn-Out an "Occupational Phenomenon": International Classification of Diseases. Available at: https://www.who.int/news/item/28-05-2019-burn-out-an-occupational-phenomenon-international-classification-of-diseases. Accessed May 15, 2021.

4. Swensen SJ. Esprit de Corps and Quality: Making the Case for Eradicating Burnout. J Healthc Manag 2018;63(1):7–11.

5. Action Collaborative on Clinician Wellbeing and Resilience. National Academy of Medicine. Available at: https://nam.edu/initiatives/clinician-resilience-and-well-being/.

6. Reith TP. Burnout in United States Healthcare Professionals: A Narrative Review. Cureus 2018;10(12):e3681.

7. Tawfik DS, Profit J, Morgenthaler TI, et al. Physician Burnout, Well-being, and Work Unit Safety Grades in Relationship to Reported Medical Errors. Mayo Clin Proc 2018;93(11):1571–80.

8. Poghosyan L, Clarke SP, Finlayson M, et al. Nurse burnout and quality of care: cross-national investigation in six countries. Res Nurs Health 2010;33(4):288–98.

9. West CP. Physician Well-Being: Expanding the Triple Aim. J Gen Intern Med 2016;31(5):458–9.

10. Sharifi M, Asadi-Pooya AA, Mousavi-Roknabadi RS. Burnout among Healthcare Providers of COVID-19; a Systematic Review of Epidemiology and Recommendations. Arch Acad Emerg Med 2020;9(1):e7.

11. Zhang XJ, Song Y, Jiang T, et al. Interventions to reduce burnout of physicians and nurses: An overview of systematic reviews and meta-analyses. Medicine (Baltimore) 2020;99(26):e20992.

12. Aryankhesal A, Mohammadibakhsh R, Hamidi Y, et al. Interventions on reducing burnout in physicians and nurses: A systematic review. Med J Islam Repub Iran 2019;33:77.

13. Moher D, Liberati A, Tetzlaff J, et al, PRISMA Group. Preferred reporting items for systematic reviews and meta-analyses: the PRISMA statement. Plos Med 2009; 6(7):e1000097.

14. Maslach C, Jackson SE, Leiter MP. Maslach burnout Inventory Manual. 4th edition. Mind Garden, Inc; 2018. Available at: https://www.mindgarden.com/117-maslach-burnout-inventory-mbi.

15. Bundy JJ, Hage AN, Srinivasa RN, et al. Burnout among interventional radiologists. J Vasc Interv Radiol 2019;31(4):1–8.

16. Campbell J, Prochazka AV, Yamashita T, et al. Predictors of persistent burnout in internal medicine residents: A prospective cohort study. Acad Med 2010;85(10): 1630–4.

17. Hyman SA, Shotwell MS, Michaels DR, et al. A survey evaluating burnout, health status, depression, reported alcohol and substance use, and social support of anesthesiologists. Anesth Analg 2017;125(6):2009–18.

18. Wells N, Shi Y, Shotwell MS, et al. Burnout and resiliency in perianesthesia nurses: Findings and recommendations from a national study of members of the American Society of PeriAnesthesia Nurses. J PeriAnesthesia Nurs 2019;34(6): 1130–45. https://doi.org/10.1016/j.jopan.2019.05.133.

19. Streu R, Hansen J, Abrahamse P, et al. Professional burnout among US plastic surgeons: Results of a national study. Ann Plast Surg 2014;72(3):346–50.

20. Card EB, Hyman SA, Wells N, et al. Burnout and resiliency in perianesthesia nurses: Findings and recommendations from a national study of members of the American Society of PeriAnesthesia Nurses. J PeriAnesthesia Nurs 2019; 34(6):1130–45. https://doi.org/10.1016/j.jopan.2019.05.133.

21. Davis S, Lind BK, Sorensen C. A comparison of burnout among oncology nurses working in adult and pediatric inpatient and outpatient settings. Oncol Nurs Forum 2013;40(4):E303–11.

22. Gallagher R, Gormley DK. Perceptions of stress, burnout, and support systems in pediatric bone marrow transplantation nursing. Clin J Oncol Nurs 2009;13(6): 681–5.

23. Gueritault-Chalvin V, Kalichman SC, Demi A, et al. Work-related stress and occupational burnout in AIDS caregivers: Test of a coping model with nurses providing AIDS care. AIDS Care 2000;12(2):149–61.

24. Meltzer LS, Missak-Huckabay L. Critical care nurses' perceptions of futile care and its effect on burnout. Am J Crit Care 2004;13(3):202–8.

25. Russell K. Perceptions of burnout, its prevention, and its effect on patient care as described by oncology nurses in the hospital setting. Oncol Nurs Forum 2016; 43(1):103–9.

26. Dyrbye LN, Varkey P, Boone SL, et al. Physician satisfaction and burnout at different career stages. Mayo Clin Proc 2013;88(12):1358–67.

27. Marchalik D, Brems J, Rodriguez A, et al. The impact of institutional factors on physician burnout: A national study of urology trainees. Urology 2019;131:27–35.

28. Ramey SJ, Ahmed AA, Takita C, et al. Burnout evaluation of radiation residents nationwide: Results of a survey of United States residents. Int J Radiat Oncol Biol Phys 2017;99(3):530–8.

29. Peery AI. Caring and burnout in registered nurses: What's the connection? Int J Hum Caring 2010;14(2):53–60.

30. Lanz JJ, Bruk-Lee V. Resilience as a moderator of the indirect effects of conflict and workload on job outcomes among nurses. J Adv Nurs 2017;73:2973–86.

31. Muir KJ, Keim-Malpass J. The emergency resiliency initiative: A pilot mindfulness intervention program. J Holist Nurs 2020;38(2):205–20.

32. Jameson BE, Bowen F. Use of the worklife and levels of burnout surveys to assess the school nurse work environment. J Sch Nurs 2020;36(4):272–82. https://doi.org/10.1177/1059840518813697.

33. Eckleberry-Hunt J, Lick D, Boura J, et al. An exploratory study of resident burnout and wellness. Acad Med 2009;84(2):269–77.

34. Rainbow JG, Steege LM. Transition to practice experiences of first- and second-career nurses: A mixed-methods study. J Clin Nurs 2019;28:1193–204. https://doi.org/10.1111/jocn.14726.

35. Attenello FJ, Buchanan IA, Wen T, et al. Factors associated with burnout among US neurosurgery residents: A nationwide survey. J Neurosurg 2018;129:1349–63.

36. Fargen KM, Arthur AS, Leslie-Mazwi T, et al. A survey of burnout and professional satisfaction among United States neurointerventionalists. J Neurointervent Surg 2019;11(11):1–6.

37. Evans R, Ghosh K. A survey of headache medicine specialists on career satisfaction and burnout. Headache 2015;55(10):1448–57. https://doi.org/10.1111/head.12708.

38. Shanafelt TD, Bradley KA, Wipf JE, et al. Burnout and self-reported patient care in an internal medicine residency program. Ann Intern Med 2002;136(5):358–67.

39. Williamson K, Lank PM, Cheema N, et al. Comparing the Maslach burnout inventory to other well-being instruments in emergency medicine residents. J Grad Med Educ 2018;10(5):532–6.

40. Lu DW, Dresden S, McCloskey C, et al. Impact of burnout on self-reported patient care among emergency physicians. West J Emerg Med 2015;16(7):996–1001.

41. West CP, Tan AD, Habermann TM, et al. Association of resident fatigue and distress with perceived medical errors. JAMA 2009;302(12):1294–300.

42. West CP, Huschka MM, Novotny PJ, et al. Association of perceived medical errors with resident distress and empathy. JAMA 2006;296(9):1071–8.

43. Adwan JZ. Pediatric nurses' grief experience, burnout and job satisfaction. J Pediatr Nurs 2014;29:329–36. https://doi.org/10.1016/j.pedn.2014.01.011.

44. Govardhan LM, Pinelli V, Schnatz PF. Burnout, depression and job satisfaction in obstetrics and gynecology residents. Conn Med 2012;76(7):389–95.

45. Shenoi AN, Kalyanaraman M, Pillai A, et al. Burnout and psychological distress among pediatric critical care physicians in the United States. Crit Care Med 2018;46(1):116–22.
46. Simons BS, Foltz PA, Chalupa RL, et al. Burnout in U.S. military orthopaedic residents and staff physicians. Mil Med 2016;181(8):835–9.
47. Messmer PR, Bragg J, Williams PD. Support programs for new graduates in pediatric nursing. J Continuing Education Nurs 2011;42(4):182–92.
48. Eckleberry-Hunt J, Kirkpatrick H, Taku K, et al. Self-report study of predictors of physician wellness, burnout, and quality of patient care. South Med J 2017; 110(4):244–8.
49. Krasner MS, Epstein RM, Beckman H, et al. Association of an educational program in mindful communication with burnout, empathy, and attitudes among primary care physicians. JAMA 2009;302(12):1284–93.
50. Mealer M, Jones J, Newman J, et al. The presence of resilience is associated with a healthier psychological profile in intensive care unit (ICU) nurses: Results of a national survey. Int J Nurs Stud 2012;49:292–9.
51. Clubbs BH, Barnette AR, Gray N, et al. A community hospital NICU developmental care partner program: Feasibility and association with decreased nurse burnout without increased infant infection rates. Adv Neonatal Care 2019;19(4): 311–20.
52. Browning L, Ryan CS, Greenberg MS, et al. Effects of cognitive adaptation on the expectation- burnout relationship among nurses. J Behav Med 2006;29(2): 139–50.
53. Doolittle BR, Windish DM, Seelig CB. Burnout, coping, and spirituality among internal medicine resident physicians. J Grad Med Educ 2013;5(2):257–61. https://doi.org/10.4300/JGME-D-12-00136.1.
54. Han S, Shanafelt TD, Sinsky CA, et al. Estimating the Attributable Cost of Physician Burnout in the United States. Ann Intern Med 2019;170(11):784–90.
55. Kelly LA, Gee PM, Butler RJ. Impact of nurse burnout on organizational and position turnover. Nurs Outlook 2021;69(1):96–102.
56. National Nursing Workforce Study. National Council of State Boards of Nursing (NCSBN). Available at: https://www.ncsbn.org/workforce.htm.

Eight Ways Nurses Can Manage a Burnt-Out Leader

Robin Squellati, PhD, APRN[a],[*],[1], George A. Zangaro, PhD, RN, FAAN[b],[2]

KEYWORDS

- Nursing • Burnout • COVID-19 • Leaders • Support

KEY POINTS

- Nurse burnout is a serious problem for America.
- The signs of a burnt-out nurse are not always easy to identify and may be physical, psychological, emotional, and/or behavioral.
- Nurses can support their peers and leaders during difficult times to reduce the effects of burnout and promote a healthy work environment.

INTRODUCTION

Nurses at all levels are leaving their jobs and the profession because of stress and burnout. Shah and colleagues found that of 50,273 US registered nurses (RNs), 31.5% left their job because of burnout.[1] This is especially alarming because the United States is facing a shortage of nurses.[2] COVID-19 added to stress and burnout in nurses, so nurses must learn to recognize and decrease the chance of burnout. The purpose of the article is to identify the signs of a burnt-out leader and strategies to effectively manage or survive in this stressful environment.

BACKGROUND

Burnout results from chronic job stress that is not well managed.[3] It is characterized as feelings of lack of energy, cynicism toward the job, decreased quality of care, and decreased professionalism.[3] Other negative effects of burnout are irritability, insomnia, and substance abuse.[4] Burnout is a work-related issue that occurs among health care professionals and may result in some people choosing to leave the

[a] Core Faculty, Walden University, Minneapolis, MN, USA; [b] American Association of Colleges of Nursing, 655 K Street NW Suite 750, Washington, DC 20001, USA
[1] Present address: 435 Chelmsford Dr, Verdi, NV 89439, USA
[2] The views, analyses, and conclusions expressed in this article are those of the authors and do not necessarily reflect the official policy or positions of the American Association of Colleges of Nursing.
* Corresponding author.
E-mail address: Robin.squellati@mail.waldenu.edu

Nurs Clin N Am 57 (2022) 67–78
https://doi.org/10.1016/j.cnur.2021.11.005
0029-6465/22/© 2021 Elsevier Inc. All rights reserved.

profession.[5] Kelly and colleagues found that all levels of nurse leaders are experiencing burnout.[6] Resiliency training and support are needed for all nurses. The factors associated with burnout need to be ameliorated to ensure an adequate supply of nurses to provide quality care to patients.

CHRONIC STRESS DURING COVID-19

Although the rate of COVID-19 hospitalizations is decreasing, one residual concern is still facing nursing. That is, the burnout rate has increased among 10,000 nurses in the *Medscape Career Satisfaction Report 2020*. Frellick reported that before COVID-19, the burnout rate for RNs was 4%, and 6 months later it was up to 18%.[7] Advanced practice registered nurses (APRNs), RNs, and licensed practical nurses (LPNs) in Frellick's study increased in burnout rates but LPNs in nursing homes felt the most burnout.[7] Of the 418,769 nurses who left their jobs in 2018, almost a third identified burnout as the reason for leaving, and 80% of those who reported burnout worked in a hospital.[8] At a time when nurses are desperately needed, precautions need to be taken to strengthen nurses and prevent burnout. COVID-19 was a stressful time for nurses and the focus now needs to turn to supporting nurses, and especially nurse leaders.

A nurse's clinical position is physically and emotionally demanding. A meta-analysis with 16 COVID-19 studies and 18,935 nurses found that the prevalence of emotional exhaustion (EE) was 34%, depersonalization (DP) was 12.6%, and feeling a lack of personal accomplishment (PA) was 15%.[9] Those at the greatest risk were younger nurses, those with less social support, and those working in a quarantine area with a high risk of contracting COVID-19. Lagasse reported that in a survey by Mental Health America, which sampled 1119 health care workers, 84% of nurses in clinical positions were at mildly burned out.[10] The ramification of this is that 48% of clinical nurses have considered retiring, quitting their present job, or changing careers.[10] Nurses leaving puts more stress on the nurse leader and remaining nurses. The nurses and leader need to work together to create a positive work situation or burnout could occur in more nurses.

During COVID-19, employers were noticing the need for intervention. Through employee assistance programs (EAPs) or health care insurance, mental health programs were offered. Some programs offered by mental health staff are stress reduction, cognitive restructuring and reframing, and grief counseling. Mental health can also help a nurse to recognize and admit to symptoms of burnout. COVID-19 was an introduction of EAPs and mental health checks that should occur routinely. Nurses will not always admit or even recognize that they need mental health support. However, if one knows the signs of burnout, they can see it in nurses.

SIGNS OF A BURNED-OUT LEADER

The signs of a burnt-out manager are not always easy to identify. The World Health Organization defines burnout as a syndrome resulting from prolonged workplace stress that is not being managed appropriately.[3] The staff nurse needs to be attentive to the signs of burnout in their leader and peers. **Table 1** provides physical, psychological, emotional, and behavioral signs of burnout. Maslach and colleagues developed the Maslach Burnout Inventory-Human Services Survey (MBI-HSS) to measure burnout in health care professionals.[11] Over the past 30 years, the MBI-HSS has become the gold standard to assess burnout in health care professionals. The instrument focuses on 3 distinct aspects of burnout: EE, DP, and PAs. Nurses who are displaying signs of exhaustion, decreased sense of accomplishment, increased DP, as well as other symptoms described in **Table 1** are likely experiencing burnout.

Table 1
Signs of burnout

Physical	Psychological	Emotional	Behavioral
Exhaustion	Fatigue	Decreased personal accomplishment	Calling in sick, arriving late, leaving early to work
Feeling tired	Difficulty concentrating	Lack of motivation	Procrastinating
Headaches	Detached from staff and family	Self-doubt	Withdrawn
Muscle tension	Decreased productivity	Cynical outlook	Intolerance to change
Decreased appetite	Decline in performance	Feeling trapped in a job	Taking frustrations out on staff
Gastrointestinal issues	Decreased creativity	Feeling alone	Increased use of alcohol
Hypertension	Negative attitude	Sense of failure	Substance misuse
Insomnia	Decreased commitment	Decreased job satisfaction	Social isolation from coworkers and family
Generalized body aches	Loss of purpose	Feeling defeated	
Weight gain	Anger, irritability		
Increased illnesses	Increased anxiety		

IMPLICATIONS OF A BURNED-OUT LEADER

A burned-out leader may experience diminished decision-making abilities, which can have negative consequences on the staff and the organization. When staff are feeling unappreciated or unsupported by their leader, they may consider other employment, which can be extremely expensive to the organization. In 2021, NSI Nursing Solutions, Inc. reported the results of a survey of hospitals across the United States and estimates the average cost of turnover for a bedside RNs is $40,038 and ranges from $28,400 to $51,700, resulting in the average hospital losing between $3.6 m and $6.5 m/y[12] The cost of turnover is staggering, and increased turnover can have a major impact on the organization's bottom line.

Another implication of burnout is an increase in absenteeism that disrupts the work environment, quality of care, innovation, employee morale, and increased hospital costs.[13] The nurse manager guides and leads staff nurses on a unit or in a department, and if the nurse manager is suffering from symptoms of burnout, this will transfer to the staff and create a poor work environment. Nurse managers are responsible for leading change and quality improvement to enhance patient outcomes, but if they are burned out, efficiency and productivity will be compromised as well as patient care and staff well-being. To ensure productivity and safe, quality patient care is being delivered, leaders in organizations must ensure that appropriate resources, both material and immaterial, are available to assist nurse managers as well as staff nurses with lessening burnout. Promoting prevention and providing appropriate support to nurse managers will significantly reduce the effects of burnout in an organization and will benefit the staff that they lead as well as the patients who are being cared for.

WAYS NURSES CAN MITIGATE THE SITUATION

Each of the suggestions below are ways to build resilience. They are a nurse's armor against stress and burnout. Nurses enjoy caring for others, but nurses also need to care for themselves and their nurse leaders. Nurses cannot control every situation and perfection is impossible with complex patients. Having a routine at work home helps one to feel more in control.[14] However, unexpected patient health situations, admissions, and a coworker getting sick can through off a routine. Talking to others may help a nurse to realize what can and cannot be accomplished and how to prioritize tasks.

STRONG INTERPERSONAL RELATIONSHIPS OUTSIDE OF WORK

Positive social interactions with a spouse, friend, or family member have the ability to reduce stress. In a large study (N = 32,417), Sørensen and colleagues found that having adequate social support modified work and nonwork stress.[15] People need a relationship where the person can talk about stressors and the listener can understand and empathize. Gallagher and colleagues found that both giving and receiving emotional support modified stress.[16] Nurses could definitely do this if they were not so tired at the end of a shift. Bryson and Bogart also found that social support helped people cope with rare diseases.[17] Nurses need family, friends, and coworkers for social and emotional support. Patients going through stressful life events required a nurse to be compassionate and caring, which becomes more difficult if the nurse is burnt-out.

WORK-LIFE BALANCE

Nurses need to balance the stress of work with fun times with family or friends. Nurses at different levels, clinical, management, or director are each affected similarly by burnout.[6] Kelly and colleagues sampled 672 nurse leaders and 2 qualitative themes emerged: the emotional drain and the negative impact on work-life balance.[6] Being intentional about setting times for friends and family is emotionally charging. Days off need to be planned to accommodate positive time. More years working as a nurse or nurse leader led to more satisfaction in the position.[6] Experience helps nurses face uncertainty. At the higher position levels, nurses had more difficulty achieving a work-life balance. With shift work, a nurse's hours are better defined, but with more administrative work, a nurse may work extra hours trying to keep up with requirements. Nurse leaders find themselves coming in early and staying late. Occasionally, nurses, including nurse leaders, should be assessed for burnout. Nurses may not want to admit to signs of burnout or even recognize how close to burnout they are feeling. A numerical score can show nurses if they are reaching burnout. Maybe some work could be shared with a coworker or discussing the workload with a supervisor may help. The boundaries between work and home may be blurred because of mission creep. Handing off assignments to junior nurses helps a junior nurse to prepare for a nurse leader role. Staff nurses need to accept committee assignments, audits, unit education, and other tasks. This is a growing opportunity and an opportunity to support nurse leaders. Nurses also have an opportunity to support each other with healthy lifestyles.

HEALTHY LIFESTYLE

A healthy lifestyle includes several components such as getting enough fluids, exercise, getting adequate sleep, and avoiding stress. Only about 25% of Americans get 6 to 8 glasses of water per day, resulting in fatigue, headaches, or difficulty focusing.[18] Aerobic exercise is another healthy activity that Americans participate in. Insufficient exercise contributes to diabetes, osteoporosis, hypertension, and arthritis.[18] Exercise also reduces stress, which is necessary to help prevent burnout.

Burnout may still occur with a healthy lifestyle but with the prevalence of burnout so high in nursing, it is important to live as healthily as possible.

Bogue and Carter created a model for nurse well-being because of the stress and burnout that nurses encounter.[19] Well-being may be enhanced with different approaches for different people, like some may focus on biophysical through adequate staffing, decreased overtime, or patient loads; some may do better with the psychoemotional by engaging with EAP, counseling, and stress management support; sociorelational by meaningful communication and inclusivity; or religiospiritual through faith services, animal therapy, or mindfulness. The sociorelational area was the strongest predictor for burnout.

Many nurses do not get enough sleep. Of those nurses in Lagasse's study, 90% said they were not getting 8 hours of sleep each night.[10] Adults need 7 to 9 hours of sleep and seniors need 7 to 8 hours.[20] Nurses have varied shifts and overtime, which may prohibit staying on a regular sleep schedule, leaving the nurse feeling continually tired.

If falling or staying asleep is a concern, talking to the primary care provider could be a first step to identifying and treating problems like breathing problems, leg cramps, or insomnia that may be associated with inadequate sleep.[20] Other tips that might help are keeping a sleep diary or using a sleep app. Symptoms of sufficient sleep include decreased reaction time, a poor attitude, poor decision-making, and ineffective communication. Nurses may need better boundaries at home to keep people and sounds from disrupting sleep time.

DECREASE STRESS

Nurses face stressors at work and home. There are toxic people and environmental situations that trigger a reaction in nurses. Some brain chemicals can help nurses to relax. Two actions that release brain chemicals, such as epinephrine, norepinephrine, serotonin, and cortisol, are relaxation breathing and laughter.[18] They seem like opposites and yet both help to reduce stress hormones, increase memory, and decrease blood pressure. Try to recall happy, positive times and times when you laughed. Make the event as colorful and vivid in your mind as possible. Write down happy remembrances as you think of them to help you when you are facing a stressful time. Then you can use these thoughts to help you decrease stress.

Nurses are under considerable stress, which may lead to burnout, no matter which type of nursing position they are in. However, oncology nurses are one type of nurses who deal with significant emotional stress. Cañadas-De la Fuente and colleagues performed a meta-analysis with 17 studies and found that oncology nurses (n = 9959) were at risk for EE and decreased PA.[4] Considering this, nurses need to encourage oncology units to participate in compassion fatigue resiliency training and a psychological skills survey for managing difficult situations. Also, at orientation and group meetings, nurses need to remind one another of the symptoms of burnout.

MINDFULNESS

Mindfulness-based interventions and self-care practices have been shown to be very effective strategies for reducing burnout and stress levels among nurses. Part of the responsibility for reducing burnout and stress rests with the organization and promoting mindfulness-based activities for the staff has been shown to be a very effective approach to reducing burnout and stress.[21,22] Activities such as meditation, stretching, and yoga are effective approaches to reducing stress and burnout in nurses. If organizations prioritize the well-being of their employees and allow them to engage in mindfulness activities to reduce stress, this will impact the care being provided in a complex health care environment.

EDUCATION

Nurses who are reporting to a burned-out manager will generally become disillusioned and burned-out. Providing education to nurses about how to manage burnout, how to recognize stress and signs of burnout will have a positive effect on the professional well-being of the nurses. Increasing awareness of burnout and implementing strategies to prevent and/or reduce stressors in the work environment will improve resilience among nurses.[23] When a nurse has specific concerns about workload or the work environment, approach the nurse manager and try to work together to reach a compromise or a solution. In some cases, nurses may determine that the only way to heal is to transition to another job either within the same organization or outside the current organization.

RECOGNIZE ACHIEVEMENTS

Leaders are motivated by significant recognition, organizational equality in rewards, and acknowledgments for a job well done.[24] However, staff nurses are also motivated by the same factors, and it is imperative that all levels of leadership and staff are appropriately recognized for achievements. The leadership in the organization should make themselves visible to the staff, conduct regular rounds to talk with nurses, and understand the stressors in the work environment that are leading to decreased engagement and productivity. The transformational leader fosters a culture of shared decision-making and seeks input from nurses at all levels in the organization to address concerns and build trust among the team. These simple approaches are cost-effective ways to decrease burnout and create a supportive and healthy work environment.

CREATE A HEALTHY WORK ENVIRONMENT

The work environment is a critical factor when assessing and/or managing burnout. A work environment where nurses feel happy/fulfilled and valued by leadership and their peers is a healthy environment where nurses are productive and engaged. Creating a culture where nurses are caring for nurses and support each other while working in a fast-paced environment is one approach to reducing burnout. Open communication, empathy, and active listening are critical to providing support to your peers. A leader may not be able to immediately remove a stressor from the environment but can provide authentic, emotional support, which can also lessen feelings of burnout. Nurse managers should also offer external support, as appropriate, through an EAP so that the employee has an outlet outside of their coworkers and family.

RECOMMENDATIONS

Nursing has done an excellent job in providing training to new graduate nurses to allow them to successfully begin their nursing career. Often, staff nurses progress to charge nurses, nurse managers, and beyond without having adequate leadership training. Leadership training is essential for all levels of nursing leadership. Kelly and colleagues found that higher levels of burnout in nurse leaders were associated with less experience in leadership, which is why nursing should ensure adequate training is provided to new and existing nurse leaders.[6] Underdeveloped leaders struggle to meet the day-to-day organizational demands and experience extreme stress while attempting to manage the staff, attend committee meetings, and be available 24/7 to support the department/unit and these issues lead to burnout.

The next generation of nurses who will be moving into leadership positions are Generation Xers and Millennials. Generation Xers were entering the workforce at a time when there were expanded career opportunities in other professions and as a result, they were less interested in a nursing career. The Millennials are surprisingly very interested in nursing and have been entering nursing at a rate almost twice that of the Baby Boomers.[25] When the Millennial generation reached age 33 years, there were almost 2 times as many who entered nursing as compared with the Generation X at an equivalent time point.[25] A major concern with the upcoming generation of leaders is the career trend that Generation Xers and Millennials will change jobs if they do not feel supported by leadership and if they are not able to maintain a quality work-life balance. These generations want to be able to have flexibility in their work schedules, control over how and when they will be at work, and desire autonomy. To effectively recruit and retain Generation X and Millennial nurses in leadership positions, current nursing leaders must consider the organizational and work-life balance factors that are important to these generations. Given the continuing need for future nurse leaders, it is critical that succession planning takes place, and the next generations of nurses are mentored and adequately prepared to assume leadership positions.

Succession planning is essential for the nursing profession because of the nursing shortage, expected retirement of baby boomers, an increase in the number of gaps in leadership positions, and the key roles nurses play in creating policy for education, practice, and nursing science.[26] Succession planning should not be solely for the purpose of filling a particular position. Leaders should identify and prepare individuals who have demonstrated leadership in their current role to be able to accept future roles within or outside of the organization. Organizational leadership must create a culture for succession planning, be willing to invest in the employees, and carefully design and implement a structured process for employees to be mentored and coached to assume new leadership roles. In health care organizations, the development of the next generation of nursing leaders is a wise business strategy because gaps in nursing leadership can have an impact on the quality of patient care, success in meeting regulatory requirements, and organizational revenue.[27]

SUPPORTING NURSE LEADERS

Burnout causes nurses to lose decision-making effectiveness and emotional intelligence may decrease.[6] The Institute for Healthcare Improvement's framework for improving "joy at work," promotes teamwork and teamwork and resilience activities. Nurses have traditionally divided workloads by patients. However, there may be other methods to divide the workload, such as having an IV nurse or an admissions nurse. If 2 nurses were working together, they may feel supported and there would be help with decision-making.

Nurses, especially informal leaders, can support their actual leaders, even if the leader has some indication burnout. Wiernikowski shows how staff nurses can offer support in several ways. One way is to understand and accept the leader's vision.[28] What does the leader see for the unit in 5 year? What improvements are required? What does the leader envision for the nursing staff? Offering constructive ideas rather than complaints or roadblocks is helpful. Another way informal leaders can support their leaders is to embrace change.[28] Instead of the common "it will not work" answer, offer to help with designing the program or policy to help ensure that nurses are successful. Informal leaders can help gather the input of as many nurses as possible to get buy-in and design a workable program.

Age is one of the key individual predictor variables in burnout.[29] In a recent meta-analysis of 51 studies, Gomez-Urquiza et al. found that older nurses reported lower

EE and DP than younger nurses, but the association of age with reduced PA was not significant.[30] Age and adequate coping skills provide protection from burnout. Older nurses can help younger nurses to learn to cope with difficult patient care situations. Older nurses could also help nurse leaders with decisions, stressful events, and dealing with difficult people.

Nurse leaders should receive education for leadership. However, many nurses earn midlevel leadership roles because they were strong and experienced clinical nurses.[6] To help leaders as well as staff nurses, the buddy system works well. Buddy up for safety, buddy for connectedness, perform buddy checks regularly, listen to a buddy, and provide hope for a buddy.[30] Buddies can help with reframing a problem, helping to find resources, and empathetic listening. At the beginning and ending of a shift, a huddle is helpful to not only go over what was done well and what could be improved but mostly to let each other know that their work was appreciated. Celebrations, thank-you notes, a flower, and candy are also ways to show appreciation.[31] Nurses can show the support of their leader in multiple ways.

Nurses need to realize that the fight is against burnout, not against the leader or other nurses. Burnout may negatively impact decision-making and critical thinking.[32] Therefore, nurses need to band together to make unit decisions, set goals, and enhance transformation. A suggestion for transforming a unit would be to study as a group to have every eligible nurse certified in their specialty. Nurses can motivate each other, intellectually stimulate each other, and celebrate accomplishments together. Another option is for nurses to join their professional organization. Finding solutions to problems becomes a shared goal. Looking through the literature, checking with others through professional organizations, and thinking outside the box stimulates nurses and transforms patient care. Poor staffing contributes to burnout, so the informal leaders need to keep up morale so that nurses are not quitting their job. A good working environment helps to decrease EE.

THERAPY

Before nurses will accept any type of therapy, a need for therapy must be realized. The Maslach Burnout Inventory (MBI) should be administered periodically to nurses. Individuals need to know and understand their scores. Based on the score, the unit may benefit from resiliency training, mindfulness training, cognitive-behavioral therapy, or another intervention. Individual scores may help nurses to realize their own potential for burnout. Awareness is needed before actions will be taken.

Preventive practices such as those previously discussed should be included. However, a healthy lifestyle may not be enough to prevent burnout. A meta-analysis by Ochentel and colleagues found that exercise was not enough to decrease burnout symptoms.[33] Combining several healthy lifestyle behaviors may increase the likelihood of reducing burnout, but other interventions may be needed.

Potard and Landais found that nurses who used negative coping strategies such as self-blame, rumination, and catastrophizing scored higher in EE and DP.[34] The goal should be for nurses to help identify when a colleague is using negative strategies. Potard and Landais found that nurses who could focus on planning, putting the problem (challenge) into proper perspective, and positive reappraisal could improve their EE and DP scores.[34] Providing educational interventions with practice to help nurses identify when a negative coping strategy is being used may be helpful. Nurses would then begin to change the negative coping strategies with positive strategies.

Bagheri and colleagues also found that positive coping strategies could decrease burnout scores.[35] Bagheri and colleagues taught stress-coping strategies and group cognitive-behavioral therapy to nurses.[35] The MBI was used to assess burnout before, immediately after training, and 1 month after training. There was significantly less burnout immediately after training and again after 1 month. Cognitive restructuring or reframing is another technique that nurses may need education and practice with.[14] Could nurses help to bring this type of training to their units? Without an intervention, some nurses will be victims of burnout.

A meta-analysis by Lee and colleagues also found that coping strategies taught to nurses could reduce burnout for at least 6 months to a year after the training.[36] Examples of coping strategies include cognitive-behavior training, stress management, mindfulness-based programs, and a team-based support group. Again, nurses need to help their leaders and each other by suggesting this type of training for the workplace. This might be linked with continuing education to help with the cost. Depression and anxiety are closely related to burnout. Those and other mental health conditions need to be handled by a professional. For nurses scoring high on the MBI, they may be encouraged to seek more testing.

FUTURE RESEARCH

Most studies on nurse burnout have been conducted with staff nurses. More research on nurse leader burnout is needed, specifically measuring burnout in nurse leaders and the factors contributing to burnout. Nurse managers' factors associated with burnout are likely very different from staff nurses and researchers should consider this comparison. Burnout is not necessarily an individual problem and future research should focus on assessing the work environment and the resiliency of the organization as well as burnout. Additional research is also needed on strategies to prevent or reduce burnout in an organization. Burnout can occur throughout an organization, and it becomes the organization's responsibility to promote and sustain a healthy work environment and reduce burnout.

The second victim phenomenon is one in which nurses and other health care providers use dysfunctional mechanisms, such as anger, projection of blame, or drugs and/or alcohol, to cope with serious mistakes in the absence of a healthier means for healing. The main purpose of this article is to provide evidence and practices that support the need for caring organizational support systems following serious adverse clinical events. Recommendations are provided on key elements of programs to prevent the prevalence, symptoms, and impact of the second victim phenomenon on our health care professionals, patients, and health care system.

SUMMARY

Rapidly increasing health care demands for an aging population, stressful hospital policies, and high-pressure work environments currently make burnout a possibility for nurse leaders. However, with mitigation, burnout does not need to be the ending of a promising nursing career. Every nurse should know the signs of burnout and continually practice methods that have demonstrated the ability to decrease burnout.

CLINICS CARE POINTS

- A vision is needed for nurses to strive for delivering the best possible patient care in a healthy work environment.
- Nurses should recognize the signs of burnout to protect each other from burnout, which results in compromised patient care.

- Nurses who face increased stress from work may find mindfulness or other actions helpful to relax and provide better patient care.
- Nurses facing burnout can evaluate their emotional exhaustion level to facilitate empathy with their patients.
- Nurses at every level should work together and share tasks to deliver optimal patient care.

DISCLOSURE

The authors have nothing to disclose.

REFERENCES

1. Shah MK, Gandrakota N, Cimiotti JP, et al. Prevalence of and factors associated with nurse burnout in the US. JAMA Netw open 2021;4(2):e2036469.
2. Zhang X, Tai D, Pforsich H, et al. United States Registered Nurse Workforce Report Card and Shortage Forecast: A Revisit. Am J Med Qual 2018;33(3):229–36.
3. World Health Organization. Burn-out an "occupational phenomenon": International Classification of Diseases. 2019. Available at: https://www.who.int/news/item/28-05-2019-burn-out-an-occupational-phenomenon-international-classification-of-diseases.
4. Cañadas-De la Fuente GA, Gómez-Urquiza JL, Ortega-Campos EM, et al. Prevalence of burnout syndrome in oncology nursing: a meta-analytic study. Psychooncology 2018;27(5):1426–33.
5. Portero de la Cruz Silvia, Cebrino Jesús, Herruzo Javier, et al. A multicenter study into burnout, perceived stress, job satisfaction, coping strategies, and general health among Emergency Department Nursing Staff. J Clin Med 2020;9(1007):1007.
6. Kelly LA, Lefton C, Fischer SA. Nurse leader burnout, satisfaction, and work-life balance. J Nurs Adm 2019;49(9):404–10.
7. Frellick M. Nurse burnout has soared during pandemic, survey shows. 2020. Available at: https://www.medscape.com/viewarticle/943091.
8. Bean M. 31% of nurses cite burnout as reason for leaving job. 2021. Available at: https://www.beckershospitalreview.com/nursing/31-of-nurses-cite-burnout-as-reason-for-leaving-job.html.
9. Galanis P, Vraka I, Fragkou D, et al. Nurses' burnout and associated risk factors during the COVID-19 pandemic: A systematic review and meta-analysis. J Adv Nurs 2021. https://doi.org/10.1111/jan.14839.
10. Lagasse J. More on workforce healthcare workers experiencing burnout, stress due to COVID-19 pandemic. Available at: https://www.healthcarefinancenews.com/news/healthcare-workers-experiencing-burnout-stress-due-covid-19-pandemic#:~:text=A%20startling%2084%25%20reported%20feeling,and%20family%20issues%20and%20responsibilities.
11. Maslach C, Jackson SE. The measurement of experienced burnout. J Occup Behav 1981;2:99–113.
12. NSI Nursing Solutions, Inc.. NSI national health care retention & RN staffing report. 2021. Available at: https://www.nsinursingsolutions.com/Documents/Library/NSI_National_Health_Care_Retention_Report.pdf.
13. Membrive-Jiménez MJ, Pradas-Hernández L, Suleiman-Martos N, et al. Burnout in nursing managers: a systematic review and meta-analysis of related factors, levels and prevalence. Int J Environ Res Public Health 2020;17(11):3983.

14. Healthcare Personnel and First Responders: How to cope with stress and build resilience during the COVID-19 pandemic. Centers for Disease Control and Prevention; 2020. Available at: https://www.cdc.gov/coronavirus/2019-ncov/hcp/mental-health-healthcare.html.

15. Sørensen JB, Lasgaard M, Willert MV, et al. The relative importance of work-related and non-work-related stressors and perceived social support on global perceived stress in a cross-sectional population-based sample. BMC Public Health 2021;21(1):543.

16. Gallagher S, O'Súilleabháin PS, Smith MA. The cardiovascular response to acute psychological stress is related to subjectively giving and receiving social support. Int J Psychophysiol 2021;164:95–102.

17. Bryson BA, Bogart KR. Social support, stress, and life satisfaction among adults with rare diseases. Health Psychol 2020;39(10):912–20.

18. Thieman L. SelfCare for HealthCare: the best way to care for patients is to care for ourselves. Nurse Leader 2018;16(6):393–7.

19. Bogue RJ, Carter KF. A model for advancing nurse well-being:: future directions for nurse leaders. Nurse Leader 2019;17(6):526–30.

20. J Perlo, B Balik, S Swensen, et al. IHI Framework for Improving Joy in Work. IHI White Paper.Cambridge, 2017 Institute for Healthcare Improvement, Cambridge, MA (2017).

21. Bianchini C, Copeland D. The use of mindfulness-based interventions to mitigate stress and burnout in nurses. J Nurses Prof Dev 2020;37(2):101–6.

22. Gilmartin H, Goyal A, Hamati MC, et al. Brief mindfulness practices for healthcare providers: a systematic literature review. Am J Med 2017;130(10):1219.e1–17.

23. Schreiber M, Cates DS, Formanski S, et al. Maximizing the resilience of healthcare workers in multi-hazard events: lessons from 2014-2015 Ebola response in Africa. Mil Med 2019;184:114–20.

24. Lewis HS, Cunningham CJL. Linking more leadership and work characteristics to nurse burnout and engagement. Nurs Res 2016;65(1):13–23.

25. Auerbach DI, Buerhaus PI, Staiger DO. Millennials almost twice as likely to be registered nurses as baby boomers were. Health Aff 2017;36(10):1804–7.

26. Branden PS, Sharts-Hopko NC. Growing clinical and academic nurse leaders: Building the pipeline. Nurs Adm Q 2017;41(3):258–65.

27. Rothwell WJ. Effective succession planning: ensuring leadership continuity and building talent from within. 5th edition. American Management Association; 2016.

28. Wiernikowski J. Leading wherever and whenever: Ensuring oncology nurses are future ready. Can Oncol Nurs J 2018;28(1):58–67. Available at: https://search-ebscohost-com.ezp.waldenulibrary.org/login.aspx?direct=true&db=rzh&AN=128130741&site=eds-live&scope=site.

29. Roche A, Ogden J. Predictors of burnout and health status in Samaritans' listening volunteers. Psychol Health Med 2017;22(10):1169–74.

30. Gómez-Urquiza JL, Vargas C, De la Fuente EI, et al. Age as a risk factor for burnout syndrome in nursing professionals: a meta-analytic study. Res Nurs Health 2017;40(2):99–110.

31. A guide to promoting health care workforce well-being during and after the COVID-19 pandemic. Boston (MA): Institute for Healthcare Improvement; 2020. Available at: www.ihi.org.

32. Wei H, King A, Jiang Y, et al. The impact of nurse leadership styles on nurse burnout: a systematic literature review. Nurse Leader 2020;18(5):439–50.

33. Ochentel O, Humphrey C, Pfeifer K. Efficacy of exercise therapy in persons with burnout. a systematic review and meta-analysis. J Sports Sci Med 2018;17(3):

475–84. Available at: https://search-ebscohost-com.ezp.waldenulibrary.org/login.aspx?direct=true&db=rzh&AN=131385250&site=eds-live&scope=site.

34. Potard C, Landais C. Relationships between frustration intolerance beliefs, cognitive emotion regulation strategies and burnout among geriatric nurses and care assistants. Geriatr Nurs 2021;42(3):700–7. Available at: https://search-ebscohost-com.ezp.waldenulibrary.org/login.aspx?direct=true&db=edo&AN=150749283&site=eds-live&scope=site.

35. Bagheri T, Fatemi MJ, Payandan H, et al. The effects of stress-coping strategies and group cognitive-behavioral therapy on nurse burnout. Ann Burns Fire Disasters 2019; 32(3):184–9. Available at: https://search-ebscohost-com.ezp.waldenulibrary.org/login.aspx?direct=true&db=mnh&AN=32313531&site=eds-live&scope=site.

36. Lee H, Chiang H, Kuo H. Relationship between authentic leadership and nurses' intent to leave: the mediating role of work environment and burnout. J Nurs Manag 2019;27(1):52–65.

Comparison of Nurse Burnout, Before and During the COVID-19 Pandemic

Debra Sullivan, PhD, MSN, RN, CNE, COI[a],*, Virginia Sullivan, MA[b],
Deborah Weatherspoon, PhD, MSN, CRNA, CNE, COI[a],
Christine Frazer, PhD, CNS, CNE[a]

KEYWORDS

- Nursing burnout • MBI • Pandemic • COVID-19 • OBI

KEY POINTS

- Nurse burnout was not well researched in past pandemics.
- The COVID-19 pandemic has seen severe rating of nurse burnout.
- Nurse burnout is a serious concern that has been correlated with negative nurse outcomes.
- There is an urgent need for health care organizations to take steps to decrease nurse burnout.

INTRODUCTION

The recent COVID-19 (also known as the coronavirus, severe acute respiratory syndrome coronavirus 2 [SARS-CoV-2]) pandemic has presented nurses with extraordinary demands in providing complex care to patients with the disease, as well as taking elaborate measures to prevent the spread of the disease to other patients, their families, and themselves.[1] These unprecedented conditions have required nurses to work longer shifts with more acute patients and limited resources, potentially leading to nurse burnout.[2] Nurse burnout has been a challenge for nurses even before the recent pandemic, but we are now seeing reports of higher levels of burnout.[3] This article looks at a history of pandemics and then examines the research of nurse burnout during previous and the current COVID-19

[a] College of Nursing, Walden University, 100 Washington Avenue South, Suite 1210, Minneapolis, MN 55401, USA; [b] General Pediatrics, Vanderbilt University Medical Center, 110 Magnolia Circle, Room 407A, Nashville, TN 37203, USA
* Corresponding author. 1581 Cunningham Road, Readyville, TN 37149.
E-mail address: Debra.sullivan@mail.waldenu.edu

Nurs Clin N Am 57 (2022) 79–99
https://doi.org/10.1016/j.cnur.2021.11.006
0029-6465/22/© 2021 Elsevier Inc. All rights reserved.

nursing.theclinics.com

pandemic. The authors conclude this article with recommendations for evidence-based interventions to decrease factors associated with nurse burnout based on our findings.

Background

Freudenberger was the first to use the term "burnout" in literature in the 1970s who defined burnout as a "state of fatigue or frustration that resulted from professional relationships that failed to produce the expected rewards."[4–6] However, nurse burnout has become a popular term and has been defined in various ways by many investigators.[4] The Maslach Burnout Inventory (MBI)[7] has widespread use as an instrument used to measure burnout.[4] Maslach[8] stated that nurses have inherently stressful jobs that can result in emotional exhaustion, depersonalization, and reduced personal accomplishment. Emotional exhaustion is defined as a "depletion of one's emotional resources and the feeling that one has nothing left to give others."[8] Depersonalization is a stage where a negative attitude toward work associates develops. The third aspect is feeling that your accomplishments do not meet personal expectations.[8] It is for this reason that Zangaro and colleagues[9] in their systematic review restricted their search of burnout to only articles that used the MBI to measure burnout in nursing. These articles in the Zangaro and colleagues'[9] systematic review spans from 2000 through 2019 and are used to investigate burnout before the COVID-19 pandemic. More recent literature is analyzed to report nurse burnout due to the COVID-19 pandemic. A recent study by the authors on nurse burnout during the COVID-19 pandemic is also discussed.

Carl Sagan said, "You have to know the past to understand the present," so in the spirit of understanding nurse burnout in the current COVID-19 pandemic, a look at literature dated before 2019 related to nurse burnout and pandemics are explored. It is essential to recognize that our population may become more prone to pandemics, as we have become a global community. The risks of spreading pathogens across geographic areas have increased.[10] Other contributing factors associated with the transmission of pathogens are cross-species transmission, climate change, and drug resistance.[10] Nurses are essential in caring for the victims of infectious disease pandemics. Nurses are traditionally vulnerable to burnout, but a pandemic increases the risk of nurse burnout, and they must be protected from burnout. High levels of nurse burnout could lead to a loss in the nursing workforce that is already experiencing an occupational shortage.[1]

PANDEMICS OF THE PAST

Pandemics have affected humans throughout histories, such as the plague, Cholera, influenza, and coronavirus diseases.[10] The Neolithic Revolution (aka, Agricultural Revolution) brought about a shift in human civilization and the way people lived.[11] A lifestyle change occurred that soon shifted from nomads hunting and gathering to large settlements of agricultural communities,[11] thereby creating prime conditions (ie, closer contact between humans and humans and animals), fostering the growth, and dispersion of pandemics.[11] Inadequate sanitation, unsafe water, and infected food supplies intensify the expansion and spread of infectious diseases throughout time. With the development of transportation systems (ships, railways, automobiles, airplanes), disease can spread more easily than at any point in history.[11]

Plagues

Looking back through history, a virus or a bacterium has caused a pandemic, and one of the first recorded pandemics was the Great Plague of Athens, dated 430 to 426 BC.[12] Falode and colleagues[12] report that this plague originated in Sudan and made its way through Egypt, across the Mediterranean into Persia and Greece. This highly contagious plague killed approximately 100,000 Athenians, as it broke out during the Peloponnesian War (431–403 BC).

During the second century AD, a period when the Roman Empire (encompassing Europe, Africa, Middle East) was thriving until a contagion, believed to be variola virus[12] (ie, smallpox), spread in the late 160s AD to Rome from Seleucia[13] following the army's return from war.[12,14] The Antonine Plague ended in 180 AD and killed 5 million people in its path.[12,15]

The first bubonic plague recorded in circa 541 to 543 AD was named the Plague of Justinian.[10,12,15] This plague differed from the previous plagues, as it was zoonotic, meaning transmission from animal to human,[12] and was caused by the bacterium Yersinia pestis.[10] Mainly found in rats and adult fleas, the bacterium is transmitted to animal hosts and between hosts, including humans when bitten by infected fleas.[10,12,15,16] Plagues can lay dormant for some time and return years later and with a vengeance. In 1345 AD the bubonic plague, known as the Black Death,[15] emerged and by 1353 AD, the worldwide death toll was 200 million, which encompassed nearly half of Europe's population.[10,11,13–15] In 1894, it emerged in China and dispersed through flea-infested rats, causing more than 12 million deaths worldwide within 10 years.[17]

As devastating as the plagues were, some positive outcomes resulted, such as institutional action to disease control, which included improved quarantine methods and better sanitation.[10,15] Scientific discoveries such as the bacillus is responsible for the plague and the culprit (fleas) in transmission by Alexandre Yersin in 1894.[10,13]

Cholera

For well over a millennium, Cholera has made its name known. This acute, and at times fatal, disease[10] began with the first wave, originating in India in 1817. After that, it got spread to other parts of the world via feces, contaminated water, or food (ie, seafood)[13] and continues to present itself, with the seventh wave occurring even until this day.[10,15] Caused by Vibrio cholerae, this has caused deaths in more than a million people.[10] In 2019, the World Health Organization (WHO)[18] estimated that 1.3 to 4 million people contact Cholera annually, and up to 143,000 deaths, caused by Cholera, occur worldwide.

Influenza

In the nineteenth, twentieth, and early twenty-first century, the WHO declared several flu pandemics. Beginning with the Russian Flu in 1889 and by most accounts ending in 1890,[13,15] this influenza virus emerged in St. Petersburg, Russia[13] and spread to large portions around the globe secondary to an increase in world population and transportation networks (ie, railways, canals, roads).[10,13,15] The worldwide fatality rate resulting from the Russian Flu is estimated at 1 million people.[10,15]

During the start of the twentieth century, The Spanish Flu emerged in 1918, and although it lasted only a year, it went down in the record books as one of the most severe pandemics in history.[11–13] Infecting an estimated 500 million people around the globe, mainly between the ages of 1 and 60 years, it had the highest impact of morbidity (50 million) occurring in the healthy young adult population (age 20–40 years).[10,13,15]

The next pandemics, both the Asian Flu (1957–1958), which originated in Singapore,[13] and the Hong Kong Flu (1968–1970), which originated in Hong Kong, involved a new strain of the influenza type A virus (H2N2 and H3N2, respectively).[10,13,15] Finally, the last influenza pandemic now known as the H1N1pdmo9, the Swine Flu (zoonotic, pigs to human, then through humans) likely originated in Mexico.

Coronavirus

The National Foundation of Infectious Diseases[19] and the Centers for Disease Control[20] report coronaviruses, named for crownlike spikes on their surface, are often circulating among animals (eg, camels, cats, and bats) and are viruses that can evolve and infect people. Coronaviruses can cause various signs and symptoms in animals and humans. For example, in cows and pigs, the virus can cause diarrhea; however, in humans it causes mild respiratory infections such as a sore throat, cough, or nasal congestion.[19,20] In the 1960s, human coronaviruses were identified.[19,20] Although there are hundreds of coronaviruses, currently only 7 human coronaviruses can affect people and can be categorized into 2 groups. The first group, common human coronaviruses, includes 229E alpha CoV, NL63 alpha CoV, OC43 beta CoV, and HKU1 beta CoV.[20] Namely, these pathogens typically cause mild upper respiratory tract infections, such as the common cold or pharyngitis.[21] The second group, known as other human coronaviruses, originated as animal infections that evolved over time and transmitted to humans.[20] These coronavirus pathogens include Middle East respiratory syndrome (MERS-CoV), SARS-CoV, and lastly, the novel coronavirus, an infectious disease representing a newly identified strain (2019-nCoV, a.k.a. SARS-CoV-2).[20,21] These pathogens also affect people and cause more severe lower respiratory tract infections/illnesses (eg, pneumonia, acute bronchitis).[21] Lastly, primary symptoms of SARS-CoV-2C are fever, shortness of breath, cough, loss of taste, or smell.[22]

To this end, history taught us that plagues, cholera, influenza, and coronavirus pandemics know no borders, and every continent, country, state, city, and community around the world are susceptible; moreover, not out of danger. Sadly, history has shown that in time pandemics repeat themselves. Looking at the lessons learned from past pandemics and taking them forward to positively affect the potential course one of them might have on the world as we know it is essential to the future of the whole human race.

RESPIRATORY PANDEMICS AND NURSE BURNOUT

Respiratory infections are especially virulent because the spread of the infectious agents are by droplets and interpersonal contact.[1] Nurses are in close contact with patients afflicted with pandemic diseases and are on the frontlines of the health care response, making them vulnerable to stressful environments.[1] Because influenza and coronavirus diseases are the most virulent, putting nurses at the highest risk, the authors discuss these pandemics and how they affect nurse burnout as reported in the literature.

Nurse Burnout Related to Influenza Pandemics

Zangaro and colleagues'[9] systematic review articles that screened articles from 2000 to 2019 for nurse burnout as measured by the entire MBI-HSS were further screened for articles related to influenza pandemics. Keywords used were "pandemic," "influenza," " Spanish flu," " avian flu," " bird flu," "Hong Kong flu," and "swine flu." This search produced no articles that met this criterion. In an attempt to find related literature, a search was then done on *Google Scholar* using the exact keywords, and only one peer-reviewed article was found related to nurse burnout. Usher and colleagues[23] addressed the H1N1 Swine flu but did not address nurse burnout, only discussing the potential to place greater demands on health services in tropical and rural regions of Australia.[23]

Coronavirus Pandemics

Coronaviruses are positive-sense, single-stranded RNA viruses and can affect humans and many species of animals.[24] Alpha-coronavirus genes are responsible for the common cold, and the beta-coronavirus causes more severe respiratory infections.[24] The beta-coronavirus includes highly pathogenic viruses that cause SAR-CoV, MERS-CoV, and SARS-CoV-2 (also known as COVID-19).[25]

The SARS-CoV was considered an epidemic and originated in Guangdong province (China) in 2003, where bats were likely responsible for passing it to humans.[26] It spread to 29 countries with 813 related fatalities.[27] MERS-CoV was reported 10 years after SARS-CoV in Saudi Arabia. It is believed that bats and camels spread the virus to humans.[28] MERS-CoV has resulted in 866 deaths in 27 countries.[27] The SARS-CoV-2 pandemic was first reported in December 2019 in Wuhan, China.[29] As of June 2021, there have been 3,899,172 deaths reported to WHO.[30]

Nurse Burnout Related to Coronavirus Pandemics

The articles in the Zangaro and colleagues'[9] systematic review were additionally filtered for coronavirus pandemics SARS-CoV, MERS-CoV, and SARS-CoV-2. Keywords used were "pandemic," "influenza," "SARS-CoV," "MERS-CoV," "SARS-CoV-19," "COVID-19," and "Coronavirus." The authors found no studies that met these criteria. A search was done on *Google Scholar* using the exact keywords but searched in years 1960 to 2021. The authors only found one article that was related to nurse burnout during SARS-CoV.

Marjanovic and colleagues'[31] was the only article found that related nurse burnout to a coronavirus pandemic before 2020. However, only the emotional exhaustion portion of the MBI was used to test for burnout, as it correlates with psychosocial variables. There were 333 nurses who were surveyed during the 2003 SAR-CoV crisis in Canada. The authors found significant positive correlations between emotional exhaustion and measures of anger, avoidance behavior, contact with patients with SARS, and time spent in quarantine. Negative correlations were found between emotional exhaustion as compared with vigor, organizational support, and trust in infection control initiatives.[31] The authors conclude that preparedness and efficacy to manage a pandemic crisis should be a priority. Teaching nurses new working strategies to prevent burnout and helping nurses reduce feelings of uncertainty and fear can benefit crisis management.[31]

Nurse Burnout Related to Current Coronavirus Pandemic

The authors then searched *Google Scholar* using keywords "nurses," pandemic," burnout," MBI," OBI," COVID-19," and " SARS-CoV-2." Combinations of keywords resulted in many narrative reviews, qualitative studies, commentaries, and study protocols, which were not considered in this report. Studies that reported statistics on burnout in nurses were included in this report (**Table 1**). Fourteen studies were found that used the MBI or portions of the MBI to report nurse burnout,[2,32–44] 1 used the Spanish Burnout Inventory,[45] 1 used the Copenhagen Burnout Inventory, and 3 used the Oldenburg Burnout Inventory (OBI).[46–48]

Table 1
Articles on nurse burnout during the COVID-19 pandemic

Article Citation	Measurement	Sample Size Nurses	Country	Setting	Findings
Lasalvia et al,[2] 2021	MBI-GS	687	NE Italy	Tertiary hospital nurses	They found that 49% of nurses displayed emotional exhaustion and were at a higher risk of burnout than other health care workers.
Huo et al,[32] 2021	MBI-GS	526	China	Frontline nurses	Researchers found that 42.5% of nurses in their study had burnout in China. Young and less experienced should receive more attention.
Wan et al,[33] 2020	MBI-GS	1011	Wuhan, China	Tertiary hospital	Found anxiety is serious but only mild to medium burnout. Note that Wuhan saw COVID-19 pneumonia patients starting in December 2019 and this study was done in February 2020 (only 2 mo later).
Lasater et al,[34] 2020	MBI-HSS	4298	US-NY and Ill	Med-Surg compared with ICU	Higher burnout in med-surg nurses (53.1%) than intensive care nurses (ICU) (46.9%). Lasater et al. pointed out that nurses working in understaffed conditions before the pandemic and understaffing conditions only worsened with the pandemic.

First author, year	Instrument	Sample size	Location	Setting	Findings
Bruyneel et al,[35] 2021	MBI-HSS	1135	Belgium	ICU	More than 68% were at risk of burnout during the first wave of COVID-19. Interestingly, this study also showed that those who perceived having a higher workload had a higher risk of burnout in all dimensions of the MBI.
Hu et al,[36] 2020	MBI-HSS	2014	Wuhan, China	Frontline nurses	Chinese version of the entire MBI-HSS was used and found that about half of the nurses reported moderate and high work burnout.
Wu et al,[37] 2020	MBI-HSS	190	Wuhan, China	Frontline compared oncology unit ward nurses	Interestingly, burnout was significantly lower in the nurses working frontline (13%) when compared with the nurses working on the unit ward (38%). The reasoning given was that perhaps frontline nurses felt more prepared with information, whereas the nurses working on the unit ward were less informed.
Guixia et al,[38] 2020	MBI-HSS	92	China	ICU compared with general ward nurses	A third study done in China found the opposite results as Wu et al. when looking at the prevalence of burnout compared with frontline ICU nurses working on general wards. An almost double number of ICU nurses (89.57%) compared general ward nurses (49.15%) with moderate to high burnout. The difference may be due to the first group working with highly vulnerable oncology patients.

(continued on next page)

Table 1
(continued)

Article Citation	Measurement	Sample Size Nurses	Country	Setting	Findings
Jose et al,[39] 2020	MBI-HSS	120	North India	ED	54% had moderate to severe levels of burnout. The researchers also found a negative correlation between burnout and resilience, in that as resilience scores were higher, burnout scores were lower.
Kakeman et al,[40] 2021	MBI-HSS	1004	Iran	Nurses who work FT in hospitals >1 y	31.5% reported "high" burnout. A positive correlation was found between emotional exhaustion and depersonalization scores and patient care quality, whereas a negative correlation was found between personal accomplishment scores and all poor care item scores. Personal accomplishment reduced the risk of occurrence of "medication errors" (OR = 0.99) and the onset of "patient and their family verbal abuse" (OR = 0.97).
Jalili et al,[41] 2021	MBI-HSS	300	Tehran, Iran	Nurses in contact with COVID-19 patients	55% experiencing high levels of burnout.

Source	Instrument	N	Setting	Location	Findings
Murat et al,[42] 2021	MBI-HSS	705	Front-line nurses at hospitals	Istanbul, Turkey	High burnout was found. "…nurses who did not feel sufficient about the nursing care experienced personal accomplishment burnout, those who worked in public hospitals and tested positive for COVID-19 experienced depersonalization burnout, and also male nurses who worked in public hospitals and tested positive for COVID-19 experienced emotional exhaustion burnout. However, it was observed that Bachelor's graduates, those who had worked for between 1 and 10 y, and nurses who did not want to work voluntarily during the pandemic had higher scores from the sub dimensions of the MBI (personal accomplishment, emotional exhaustion, depersonalization); in other words, they were more negatively affected."
Galanis et al,[43] 2021	MBI-HSS	18,935	Systematic review of 16 articles	China, Turkey, Italy, Singapore, Puerto Rico, UK, India, Iran, Spain, Japan, USA, Spain	Nurses working during COVID-19 pandemic. Overall, the study reported emotional exhaustion was 34.1%, depersonalization was 12.6%, and lack of personal accomplishment was 15.2%. High scores on emotional exhaustion (>20) and depersonalization (>10) and low scores on personal accomplishment (<25) indicate burnout. (Maslach et al., 1996).

(continued on next page)

Table 1
(continued)

Article Citation	Measurement	Sample Size Nurses	Country	Setting	Findings
					These findings would be in agreement with most of the conclusions of the articles reviewed here.
Prasad et al,[44] 2021	MBI-one question	5027	US	Nurses working during COVID-19 pandemic	A national survey only asked one question from the MBI about burnout and found 53.87% had burnout
Garcia et al,[45] 2021	Spanish Burnout Inventory	771	Spain	Nurses working in hospitals during COVID-19 pandemic	"The perceived threat of COVID-19 positively correlates with burnout (0.68; $P < .01$). This correlation is the highest between burnout and the variables used to explain it"
Chor et al,[53] 2020	Copenhagen Burnout Inventory	210	Singapore	ED and urgent care nurses	53.3% were experiencing burnout during the pandemic.
Hoseinabadi et al,[46] 2020	OBI	245	Iran	151 frontline nurses compared with 94 nurses not exposed to COVID-19 patients	Frontline nurses scored 2.57 out of 5 and nonexposed nurses scored 2.51
Horta et al,[47] 2021	OBI	123	Brazil	Frontline nurse	60% were exhausted, with 41% experiencing burnout.

| Bellanti et al,[48] 2021 | MBI
OBI | 293 | Italy | Frontline nurses | This study compared the MBI scores with OBI scores. The MBI reported moderate/high emotional exhaustion in 76.5%, depersonalization in 50.2%, and personal gratification in 54.6% of participants. Compared with the OBI, which resulted in medium/high burnout in 89.1% of participants.[48] Pearson's correlations of the MBI and OBI and the sub-dimensions found exhaustion detected by MBI or OBI showed 50% agreement, with 197 (67.2%) of participants with a high level of exhaustion on both tools. |

Abbreviations: GS, General Survey; HSS, Human Services Survey; MBI, Maslach Burnout Inventory; OBI, Oldenburg Burnout Inventory.

Based on these findings, nurse burnout was not well researched during past pandemics. However, there is evidence that nurse burnout is moderate to high under normal circumstances. Current research does show overwhelming evidence that nurse burnout has increased during the COVID-19 pandemic.

PRELIMINARY RESULTS OF A STUDY ON NURSE BURNOUT DURING COVID-19

In this section, the authors report on their own cross-sectional, online survey study preliminary findings. This study was carried out from April 7, 2020, to January 15, 2021, when COVID-19 first hit the United States. Included are data from nurses in 48 states (no data were obtained from nurses in Utah and Alaska) and 2 other countries. The purpose of this study was to examine the mental health of nurses during the COVID-19 pandemic. It was hypothesized that there would be higher rates of adverse mental health outcomes due to staffing shortages, increased stress due to the fear of contracting COVID-19, and low amounts of support and protection, among other reasons. Participants in this study were administered several standardized measures of 4 aspects of mental health (depression, anxiety, trauma, and burnout) via an online survey. The finding from the burnout measure will be reported in the following discussion.

In the authors' study the Oldenburg Burnout Inventory (OBI)[49] was administered to measure nurse burnout, as it is a free public domain instrument. It has been validated as a reliable instrument.[50,51] In their study, the OBI was administered to 1364 nurses working during the COVID-19 pandemic as part of this online survey. The OBI is a 16-item measure of 2 dimensions of burnout scored by a 4-point scale ranging from 1 (strongly agree) to 4 (strongly disagree). All scores were reversed (except for reverse scoring items) so that higher scores indicated more burnout. The OBI measures 2 dimensions of burnout, exhaustion, and disengagement from work. These 2 dimensions have been found to have a moderate-to-high correlation with the emotional exhaustion and depersonalization scales of the Maslach Burnout Inventory ($r = .716$ and $r = .550$, respectively) (Bellanti). For this analysis, a cutoff score of greater than or equal to 2.25 was used to determine exhaustion on the OBI, and a cutoff score of greater than or equal to 2.1 was used to determine disengagement on the OBI, as recommended by Peterson and colleagues[52] in their study on 3719 health care workers.

The authors removed 327 participants from this dataset due to partial or incomplete OBI scores ($n = 1037$). Demographics for the 1037 nurses are listed as follows:

- The participants were 92% women and 8% men
- Highest percentage of age groups were 55 to 64 years at 27%, 45 to 54 years at 24%, and 35 to 44 years at 21%.
- Highest degree earned: Associate Degree 17%, BSN 52%, Masters 25%, Doctorate 6.7%
- 39% were nursing students
- Employment: clinic was 11%, hospital was 55%, and other 34%
- Location of hospital: urban 55%, suburban 32%, rural 14%
- Location of residence: urban 17%, suburban 56%, rural 27%
- Participants were represented from every US state except Alaska.
  - 1 participant from Puerto Rico
  - Top 2 states represented was Florida with 19% and New York with 18%
- International participants included: Canada 4, United Kingdom 2, and one from each of the following countries: Bahamas, Nepal, South Africa, South Korea, United Republic of Tanzania, and Zimbabwe.

Based on these recommended cutoff scores, we found that 705 (68.0%) nurses in this dataset met the criteria for the exhaustion dimension of burnout, and 916 (88.3%) nurses met the criteria for the disengagement dimension of burnout. To further examine contributors to burnout in nurses during the COVID-19 pandemic, we correlated the burnout scores with demographic variables, asking whether the nurse was working on the frontlines of the pandemic and a set of questions about possible contributing factors to burnout during the pandemic. Because of the nature of the response options for some questions, Spearman's r was calculated instead of Pearson's r. All statistical tests use a .05 significance, and all were done in a two-tailed fashion. Responses to these questions were not required for participation, and therefore, not all participants who completed the OBI completed the demographics, frontline question, or contributing factors questions. The varied responses led to different sample sizes for these questions; these n values are shown in the last column of the following tables.

Results from the demographic variables and the full-scale OBI are presented in **Table 2**. Significant, negative correlations were found for age, education, and level of contact with patients with COVID-19 (frontline workers). A significant, positive correlation was identified between burnout and whether or not the nurse is a current degree-seeking student. Based on Cohen's recommendations for the strength of a correlation, the demographic variable "age" showed a weak, negative correlation ($r = -.298$).[54] However, although other variables were significant, they were not strong relationships, according to these recommendations.[54]

Near the end of the online survey, we asked a series of questions related to possible contributing factors to mental health and burnout, specific to the pandemic. For the full-scale OBI, we found positive, significant correlations for the first question, "Estimate what capacity your hospital is at right now" (capacity), the second question, "Do you feel that there is a shortage of personal protective equipment (PPE) at your hospital?" (PPE), and the fifth question "Are you working overtime due to the COVID-19 pandemic?" (overtime). We found negative, significant correlations for the third question "How staffed do you feel your institution is?" (staffed feel), the fourth question "Do you feel that your institution is adequately staffed?" (staffed adequate), and the eighth question "Do you feel that you are being adequately paid for your work?"(adequate pay). Based on Cohen's recommendations for the strength of a correlation, questions 3 (staffed feel), 4 (staffed adequate), and 8 (adequate pay) showed weak, negative correlations ($r = -.304$, $r = -.266$, and $r = -.280$, respectively).[54]

The authors also examined the association between these questions and the exhaustion and disengagement subscales of the OBI (**Table 3**). They found significant,

Table 2
Correlations between full-scale Oldenburg Burnout Inventory and demographic variables

Demographic Variable	Spearman's r_s	P-value	n
Age	$-.298^a$	.000	1036
Gender	.026	.413	1032
Education	$-.081^a$	.009	1034
Current Student	$.142^a$	.000	1031
Marital Status	.061	.051	1037
Level of contact with COVID-19 patients/ frontline worker	$-.170^a$	.000	1037

Bold values are significant.
[a] Significant at the .001 level.

Table 3
Correlations between contributing factors during the COVID-19 pandemic and burnout

Hospital Measure	Spearman's rs	P-value	n
Full-Scale			
1. Estimate what capacity your hospital is at right now.	.073[a]	.033	855
2. Do you feel that there is a shortage of personal protective equipment (PPE) at your hospital?	.224[b]	<.001	810
3. How staffed do you feel your institution is?	−.304[b]	<.001	921
4. Do you feel that your institution is adequately staffed?	−.266[b]	<.001	835
5. Are you working overtime due to the COVID-19 pandemic?	.172[b]	<.001	980
6. Estimate how many hours of overtime you are working.	.077	.157	338
7. Are you being paid overtime wages for your overtime work?	.035	.519	334
8. Do you feel that you are being adequately paid for your work?	−.280[b]	<.001	869
Exhaustion			
1. Estimate what capacity your hospital is at right now.	.095[a]	.006	855
2. Do you feel that there is a shortage of personal protective equipment (PPE) at your hospital?	.234[b]	<.001	810
3. How staffed do you feel your institution is?	−.293[b]	<.001	921
4. Do you feel that your institution is adequately staffed?	−.254[b]	<.001	835
5. Are you working overtime due to the COVID-19 pandemic?	.205[b]	<.001	980
6. Estimate how many hours of overtime you are working.	.078	.150	338
7. Are you being paid overtime wages for your overtime work?	.031	.577	334
8. Do you feel that you are being adequately paid for your work?	−.251[b]	<.001	869
Disengagement			
1. Estimate what capacity your hospital is at right now.	.042	.216	855
2. Do you feel that there is a shortage of personal protective equipment (PPE) at your hospital?	.180[b]	<.001	810
3. How staffed do you feel your institution is?	−.265[b]	<.001	921

4. Do you feel that your institution is adequately staffed?	**−.238**[b]	< .001	835
5. Are you working overtime due to the COVID-19 pandemic?	**.115**[b]	< .001	980
6. Estimate how many hours of overtime you are working.	.073	.183	338
7. Are you being paid overtime wages for your overtime work?	.043	.432	334
8. Do you feel that you are being adequately paid for your work?	**−.259**[b]	< .001	869

Bold values are significant.
[a] Significant at the .05 level.
[b] Significant at the .001 level.

positive correlations between questions 1 (capacity), 2 (PPE), and 5 (overtime work) and the exhaustion subscale. Significant, negative correlations between the exhaustion subscale and questions 3 (staffed feel), 4 (staffed adequate), and 8 (adequate pay) were identified. Significant, positive correlations were found between questions 2 (PPE) and 5 (overtime work) and the disengagement subscale. Significant, negative correlations between the disengagement subscale and questions 3 (staffed feel), 4 (staffed adequate), and 8 (adequate pay) were identified. Based on Cohen's recommendations, questions 3 (staffed feel), 4 (staffed adequate), and 8 (adequate pay) showed weak, negative correlations with the exhaustion subscale ($r = -.293$, $r = -.254$, and $r = -.251$, respectively), and questions 3 (staffed feel) and 8 (adequate pay) showed weak, negative correlations with the disengagement subscale ($r = -.265$ and $r = -.259$, respectively).[54] These results are similar to the findings for the full-scale OBI, and these findings are discussed in terms of overall burnout. Because of the nature of the scoring of this scale, the authors thought it was beneficial to observe these relationships in terms of these subscales as well.

Weak, negative associations were found between the questions 3 (staffed feel) and 4 (staffed adequate) and 8 (adequate pay). Nurses working during the COVID-19 pandemic who felt that their institution was more staffed experienced less burnout than those who reported that their institution was understaffed. Likewise, nurses who felt that their institution was adequately staffed were less burned out than those who felt that their institution was not adequately staffed. Lastly, nurses who felt that they were adequately paid for their work during the COVID-19 pandemic were experiencing less burnout, and those who did not feel that they were adequately paid were more burned out. Adequate hospital staffing is an environmental stressor that has been shown to affect burnout in nurses in several other studies.[55] It was expected that there is a more robust correlation during the COVID-19 pandemic, but these results show that adequate staffing is a problem for nurse burnout during the COVID-19 pandemic. Another study that investigated pay and burnout found that wage was associated with job dissatisfaction and intent to leave but only had a small effect on burnout.[56] The relationship between pay and burnout in this study is weak, but it suggests that nurses who do not feel they are being adequately paid for the increase in work due to the pandemic experience more burnout.

SUMMARY

Global pandemics present a unique challenge to nurses who already show high rates of burnout.[57] This topic is of considerable interest at the present time because of the incredible demand that has been placed on nurses during the COVID-19 pandemic. In the authors' literature review, they found that nurses experience high rates of burnout when working under normal circumstances, but even higher rates of burnout are being reported during the COVID-19 pandemic.[2] In a study conducted by the authors of this article, nurses are experiencing high rates of burnout during the COVID-19 pandemic. The 2 dimensions measured by the OBI have moderate to high correlations with the emotional exhaustion and depersonalization scales of the MBI ($r = 0.716$ and $r = 0.550$, respectively).[49] The MBI is considered the "gold standard" tool for measuring burnout and was used in several studies mentioned in this article, where high rates of burnout are also reported.[2,32–44] In the authors study, 68.0% of nurses met criteria for the exhaustion dimension, and 88.3% of nurses met criteria for the depersonalization dimension.

In the study conducted by the authors of this article, there were some contributing factors to burnout, which other studies have supported, such as job stress,[44,46,48] inadequate staffing,[34] and inadequate pay for the work performed.[56] However, the findings from the authors' study are even higher than has been reported in other studies. When combined with findings from other studies, these results provide evidence that nurses need additional support during global pandemics to decrease burnout and combat its adverse consequences, such as poor quality of patient care, nurse turnover, and negative consequences for the nurse's health.

Literature has suggested that health care organizations can support their nurses and lower burnout by addressing these factors and creating policies to protect nurses.[34,36] Health care organizations should monitor nurses for risk of burnout.[35,58–60] Studies performed during the COVID-19 pandemic and other pandemics have found various ways to support nurses and decrease burnout such as teaching nurses new strategies to protect their well-being.[1,60,61] These strategies include mindfulness training,[60,62,63] self-care techniques,[40] access to psychosocial and psychological support,[40,42,47,48] prioritizing rest and breaks,[47] and meditation apps.[62] Preventing burnout and supporting nurses to reduce feelings of uncertainty and fear[32] can benefit crisis management during pandemics.[31,64]

In conclusion, this literature review and the authors' research confirmed that nurses are experiencing high levels of burnout during the COVID-19 pandemic and suggest that health care organizations need to support nurses by creating policies to protect nurses, monitoring nurses for signs and symptoms of burnout, and helping nurses to implement strategies to protect their well-being.

CLINICS CARE POINTS

- Health care organizations should support nurses by implementing interventions to protect their well-being.
- Nurses should be monitored for risk of burnout.
- Policies should be written to protect nurses from inadequate staffing and prioritizing rest and breaks.

DISCLOSURE

The authors have nothing to disclose.

REFERENCES

1. Fernandez R, Lord H, Halcomb E, et al. Implications for COVID-19: a systematic review of nurses' experiences of working in acute care hospital settings during a respiratory pandemic. Int J Nurs Stud 2020;111:103637.
2. Lasalvia A, Amaddeo F, Porru S, et al. Levels of burn-out among healthcare workers during the COVID-19 pandemic and their associated factors: a cross-sectional study in a tertiary hospital of a highly burdened area of north-east Italy. BMJ Open 2021;11:e045127.
3. Kok N, van Gurp J, Teerenstra S, et al. Coronavirus disease 2019 immediately increases burnout symptoms in ICU professionals: a longitudinal cohort study. Crit Care Med 2021;49(3):419–27.
4. Poghosyan L, Aiken LH, Sloane DM. Factor structure of the Maslach burnout inventory: an analysis of data from large scale cross-sectional surveys of nurses from eight countries. Int J Nurs Stud 2009;46(7):894–902 [Erratum appears in Int J Nurs Stud. 2014 Oct;51(10):1416-7].

5. Freudenberger HJ. Staff burnout. J Soc Issues 1974;30:159–65.
6. Freudenberger HJ, Richelson GI. Burn-out: the high cost of high achievement. New York: Anchor Pres, Doubleday & Company, Inc; 1980.
7. Maslach C, Jackson SE. The measurement of experienced burnout. J Organ Behav 1981;2:99–113.
8. Maslach C. Burnout: the cost of caring. Englewood Cliffs (NJ): Prentice Hall; 1982.
9. Zangaro G, Dulko D, Sullivan D, et al. Systematic review of bunout in U.S. nurses. 2022: In print.
10. Piret J, Boivin G. Pandemics throughout history. Front Microbiol 2021;11:631736.
11. Moore J. Pandemics and plagues: teaching history's biggest killers. Ohio Social Stud Rev 2020;56(2):5–21. Avalable at: https://ossr.scholasticahq.com/article/17365-pandemics-and-plagues-teaching-history-s-biggest-killers. Accessed July 1, 2021.
12. Falode A, Yakubu M, Bolarinwa O. History of pandemics in the twentieth and twenty-first century. Sineza 2021;2(1):9–26.
13. Turner JA. Pandemics and epidemics through history: this too shall pass. J Hosp Librariansh 2020;20(3):280–7.
14. Bower B. Past plagues offer lessons for society: starting with the Roman Empire, societies have often been resilient through deadly outbreaks. Sci News 2020; 197(11):24–7. Available at: https://www.sciencenews.org/article/coronavirus-covid-19-ancient-plagues-pandemics-lessons-society. Accessed July 1, 2021.
15. Dasgupta S, Crunkhorn R. A history of pandemics through the ages and the human cost. The Physician 2020;6(2):1–9.
16. Ditchburn J-L, Hodgkins R. Yersinia pestis, a problem of the past and a re-emerging threat. Biosaf Health 2019;1(2):65–70.
17. World Health Organization [WHO]. WHO report on global surveillance of epidemic-prone infectious diseases. Available at: https://www.who.int/csr/resources/publications/surveillance/plague.pdf. Accessed July 1, 2021.
18. World Health Organization [WHO]. Cholera fact sheet. Available at: https://www.who.int/news-room/fact-sheets/detail/cholera. Accessed July 5, 2021.
19. National Foundation of Infectious Diseases. Coronaviruses. Available at: https://www.nfid.org/infectious-diseases/coronaviruses/.
20. Centers for Disease Control [CDC]. Human coronavirus types. Available at: https://www.cdc.gov/coronavirus/types.html. Accessed July 6, 2021.
21. Liu DX, Liang JQ, Fung TO. Human Coronavirus-229E, -OC43, -NL63, and -HKU1 (Coronaviridae). Encyclopedia Virol 2021;3:428–40.
22. Center for Disease Control. [CDC]. Symptoms of COVID-19. Available at: https://www.cdc.gov/coronavirus/2019-ncov/symptoms-testing/symptoms.html. Accessed July 5, 2021.
23. Usher K, Gardner A, Buttner P, et al. The H1N1 influenza 09 and its potential impact on the Australian nursing workforce. Collegian 2009;16(4):169–70.
24. Kahn JS, McIntosh K. History and recent advances in coronavirus discovery. Pediatr Infect Dis J 2005;24:S223–7 [discussion: S226].
25. Song Z, Xu Y, Bao L, et al. From SARS to MERS, thrusting coronaviruses into the spotlight. Viruses 2019;11:59.
26. Guan Y, Zheng BJ, He Y, et al. Isolation and characterization of viruses related to the SARS coronavirus from animals insouthern China. Science 2003;302(276):276–8.

27. World Health Organization [WHO]. Cumulative number of reported probable cases of SARS. 2oo3. Available at: https://www.who.int/news-room/fact-sheets/detail/plague.

28. Conde R, Grant R, Malik MR, et al. Reported direct and indirect contact with dromedary camels among laboratory-confirmed MERS-CoV cases. Viruses 2018;10:425.

29. Lau SKP, Luk HKH, Wong ACP, et al. Possible bat origin of severe acute respiratory syndrome coronavirus 2. Emerg Infect Dis 2020;26:1542–7.

30. World Health Organization [WHO]. WHO Coronavirus Disease (COVID-19) Dashboard. 2021. Available at: https://covid19.who.int/. Accessed July 19, 2021.

31. Marjanovic Z, Greenglass ER, Coffey S. The relevance of psychosocial variables and working conditions in predicting nurses' coping strategies during the SARS crisis: An online questionnaire survey. Int J Nurs Stud 2007;44(6):991–8.

32. Huo L, Zhou Y, Li S, et al. Burnout and its relationship with depressive symptoms in medical staff during the COVID-19 epidemic in China. Front Psychol 2021;12:616369.

33. Wan Z, Lian M, Ma H, et al. Factors associated with burnout among Chinese nurses during COVID-19 epidemic: a cross sectional study. Res Square 2020. https://doi.org/10.21203/rs.3.rs-31486/v1.

34. Lasater KB, Aiken LH, Sloane DM, et al. Chronic hospital nurse understaffing meets COVID-19: an observational study. BMJ Qual Saf 2020;0:1–9.

35. Bruyneel A, Smith P, Tack J, et al. Prevalence of burnout risk and factors associated with burnout risk among ICU nurses during the COVID-19 outbreak in French speaking Belgium. Intensive Crit Care Nurs 2021;65:103059.

36. Hu D, Kong Y, Li W, et al. Frontline nurses's burnout, anxiety, depression, and fear statuses and their associated factors during the COVID-19 outbreak in Wuhan, China: A large-scal cross-sectional study. EClinicalMedicine 2020;24:100424.

37. Wu Y, Wang J, Luo C, et al. A comparison of burnout frequency among oncology physicians and nurses working on the frontline and usual wards during the COVID-19 Epidemic in Wuhan, China. J Pain Symptom Manage 2020;60(1):e60–5.

38. Guixia L, Hui Z. A Study on burnout of nurses in the period of COVID-19. Psychol Behav Sci 2020;9(3):31–6.

39. Jose S, Dhandapani M, Cyriac MC. Burnout and resilience among frontline nurses during COVID-19 pandemic: A cross-sectional study in the emergency department of a tertiary care center, North India. Indian J Crit Care Med 2020;24(11):1081–8.

40. Kakemam E, Chegini A, Rouhi A, et al. Burout and its relationship to self-reported quality of patient care and adverse events during COVID-19: A cross-sectional online survey among nurses. J Nurs Manag 2021;00:1–9.

41. Jalili M, Niroomand M, Hadavand F, et al. Burnout among healthcare professionals during COVID-19 pandemic: a crosss-sectional study. Int Arch Occup Environ Health 2021. https://doi.org/10.1007/s00420-021-01695-x.

42. Murat M, Kose S, Savaser S. Determination of stress, depression and burnout levels of front-line nurses during the COVID-19 pandemic. Int J Ment Health Nurs 2021;30:533–43.

43. Galanis P, Vraka I, Fragkou D, et al. Nurses' burnout and associated risk factors during the COVID-19 pandemic: A systematic review and meta-analysis. J Adv Nurs 2021;77(8):3286–302.

44. Prasad K, McLoughlin C, Stillman M, et al. Prevalence and correlates of stress and burnout among U.S. healthcare workers during COVID-19 pandemic: A national cross-sectional survey study. EClinicalMedicine 2021;35:100879.

45. Garcia GM, Calvo JCA. The threat of COVID-19 and its influence on nursing staff burnout. J Adv Nurs 2021;77:8323–844.

46. Chor WPD, Ng WM, Cheng L, et al. Burnout amongst emergency healthcare workers during COVID-19 pandemic: a multi-center study. Am J Emerg Med 2020. https://doi.org/10.1016/j.ajem.2020.10.040.

47. Hoseinabadi TS, Kakhki S, Teimori G, et al. Burnout and its influencing factors between frontline nurses and nurses from other wards during the outbreak of Coronavirus Disease (COVID-19) in Iran. Invest Educ Enferm 2020;38(2):e03.

48. Horta RL, Camargo EG, Barbosa MLL, et al. Front line staff nurses and mental health during COVID-19 pandemic in a general hospital. J Bras Psiquiatr 2021; 70(1). https://doi.org/10.1590/0047-2085000000316.

49. Bellanti F, Lo Buglio A, Capuano E, et al. Factors related to nurses' burnout during the first wave of Coronavirus Disease-19 in a University Hospital in Italy. Int J Environ Res Public Health 2021;18(10):5051.

50. Demerouti E, Bakker AB, Vardakou I, et al. The convergent validity of two burnout instruments: A multitrait-multimethod analysis. Eur J Psychol Assess 2003;19: 12–23.

51. Demerouti E, Mostert K, Bakker AB. Burnout and work engagement: a thorough investigation of the independency of both constructs. J Occup Health Psychol 2010;15(3):209–22.

52. Demerouti E, Veldhuis W, Coombes C, et al. Burnout among pilots: psychological factors related to happiness and performance at simulator training. Ergonomics 2018. https://doi.org/10.1080/00140139.2018.1464667.

53. Peterson U, Demerouti E, Bergström G, et al. Burnout and physical and mental health among Swedish healthcare workers. J Adv Nurs 2008;62(1):84–95.

54. Cohen J. Statistical power analysis for the behavioral sciences. Burlington (MA): Elsevier Science; 2013.

55. Aiken LH, Clarke SP, Sloane DM. International Hospital Outcomes Research Consortium. Hospital staffing, organization, and quality of care: cross-national findings. Int J Qual Health Care 2002;14(1):5–14.

56. McHugh MD, Ma C. Wage, work environment, and staffing: effects on nurse outcomes. Policy Polit Nurs Pract 2014;15(3–4):72–80.

57. Bradley M, Chahar P. Burnout of healthcare providers during COVID-19. Cleve Clin J Med 2020. https://doi.org/10.3949/ccjm.87a.ccc051.

58. Weilenmann s, Ernst J, Petry H. Healthcare workers' mental health during the first weeks of SARS-CoV-2 pandemic in Switzerland-A cross -sectional study. Front Psychol 2021;12:594340.

59. Ross J. The exacerbation of burnout during COVID-19: A major concern for nurse safety. J Post Anesth Nurs 2020;35(4):439–40.

60. Tunaiji HA, Qubaisi MA, Dalkilinc M, et al. Impact of COVID-19 pandemic burnout on cardiovascular risk in healthcare professionals study protocol: A multicenter exploratory longitudinal study. Front Psychol 2020;22:571057.

61. Kealy A. While U.S. nurses fight COVID-19 in hospitals they also fight burnout. J Health Care Finance 2020. Available at: www.HealthFinanceJournal.com. Accessed July 10, 2021.

62. Janeway D. The role of psychiatry in treating burnout among nurses during COVID-19 pandemic. J Radiol Nurs 2020;39:176–8.

63. Luberto CM, Goodman JH, Halvorson B, et al. Stress and coping among health professions students during COVID-19: A perspective on the benefits of mindfulness. Glob Adv Health Med 2020;9:1–5.

64. Okediran JO, Ilesanmi OS, Fetuga AA, et al. The experiences of healthcare workers during the COVID-19 crisis in Lagos, Nigeria: A qualitative study. Germs 2020;10(4):356–66.

How Do We Reduce Burnout In Nursing?

Dorothy Dulko, PhD, ARNP-BC, AOCNP, WHNP-BC[a,1,*], Betty J. Kohal, DNP, PMHCNS-BC[b]

KEYWORDS

- Nurse burnout • Residencies • Preceptors • Mindfulness • Gratitude
- Compassion satisfaction

KEY POINTS

- Burnout has reached concerning levels among US health care professionals, with one-third of nurses reporting symptoms.
- Patient safety fears, workplace incivility, and poor communication with colleagues contribute to professional dissatisfaction and nurse burnout.
- Organizational support, training, and professional development opportunities are imperative for novice and experienced nurses.
- High levels of compassion satisfaction appear to have an inverse relationship with burnout.

INTRODUCTION

Burnout syndrome has been defined by Maslach and colleagues[1] as a state of chronic stress characterized by high levels of emotional exhaustion and depersonalization and low levels of professional efficacy. Burnout is described within 3 dimensions: (a) feelings of energy depletion or exhaustion; (b) increased mental distance from one's job; and (c) reduced professional efficacy.[2]

Burnout has reached concerning levels among US health care professionals, with more than one-third of nurses reporting symptoms.[3] The effects of nurse burnout include poor job satisfaction, moral distress, and turnover.[4] Although the relationship between an individual nurse and their health care organization may differ based on the nurse's level of experience, there is little research that explores the relationship between experience level, organization environment, and nurse burnout.

Nurses' physical well-being and mental well-being are both essential to sustaining a healthy nursing workforce. Factors such as an empowering work environment have

[a] American Association of Colleges of Nursing, 655 K Street, NW, Suite 750 Washington, DC 20001, USA; [b] Walden University, College of Nursing, 100 Washington Avenue South, Suite 1210, Minneapolis, MN 55401, USA
[1] The views, analyses, and conclusions expressed in this article are those of the authors and do not necessarily reflect the official policy or positions of the American Association of Colleges of Nursing.
* Corresponding author.
E-mail address: dorothydulko@gmail.com

Nurs Clin N Am 57 (2022) 101–114
https://doi.org/10.1016/j.cnur.2021.11.007
0029-6465/22/© 2021 Elsevier Inc. All rights reserved.
nursing.theclinics.com

shown positive effects on nurses' mental health.[5] Formal and informal individual and organizational approaches to support nurse transition and sustained practice fulfillment are key to successful integration into professional nursing roles and ensuring ongoing retention.[6]

Although many health care organizations enjoy relationships with colleges of nursing supporting a recruitment pipeline of new graduate nurses, engaging and retaining nurses on a long-term basis remain challenging. Attention to the well-being of novice nurses is not only vital to nurse retention overall but also essential to patient satisfaction and outcomes.[7] Discouraging experiences, such as not feeling respected or appreciated, unrealistic workload, and lateral nurse bullying, are frequently reported reasons for nurses leaving their positions.[8] This, coupled with caustic communications with health care colleagues, including physicians, results in many nurses reconsidering their chosen profession entirely.[9]

A collaborative research project at Indiana University Health Ball Memorial Hospital, including a nurse scientist, associate professor of nursing, clinical nurse specialist, direct care nurse, nurse educator, and chief nursing officer, found that nurses reported low job satisfaction related to heavy workloads and often felt unable to ensure patient safety.[10] Disillusionment related to schedules, relationships with peers, autonomy, and insufficient time with patients were reported, with discontent peaking between 4 and 6 months and again near the end of the second year of practice. This research frames future study of academic-clinical practice partnerships, the need for deeper collaborations between nursing faculty and nurse leaders within health care organizations, and the potential importance of nurse residencies for new graduate nurses.

Organizational approaches to role transition, self-confidence building, and empowerment are essential to reducing nurse burnout and successful nurse retention. It is imperative for health care organizations to understand the prevalence, predictors, barriers, and facilitators of nurse well-being and professional quality of life.[11]

NATURE OF THE PROBLEM: BURNOUT

At more than 6 million in 2019, nurses represent the largest number of professionals in the health care workforce, with nurses comprising nearly 30% of hospital employees in the United States.[12] Nurses frequently describe finding the initial 1 to 2 years of practice to be especially challenging and stressful,[13] reporting high levels of anxiety, stress, and burnout during their initial years in the workforce.[14] Many nurses consider leaving the profession in their first 2 to 5 years of practice,[15] with younger nurses, under age 40, appearing to experience burnout at a higher rate.[16] In 2020, the median age of registered nurses was 52 years, up from 51 years in 2017. Nurses aged 65 years or older accounted for 19% of the workforce, up from 14.6% in 2017 and 4.4% in 2013.[17] The aging of the nurse workforce represents an imperative to both recruit and retain novice and younger nurses.

Commonly reported causes of nurses' intention to leave their positions include feelings of incompetence, lateral "nurse-to-nurse" violence, and poor interdisciplinary relationships with other health care professionals, such as physicians.[17] There is increasing evidence that workplace incivility is prevalent in nursing, with research supporting that nearly 30% of nurses experience bullying within the first 6 months of their nursing career.[18] Burnout, bullying, and workplace incivility have been associated with poor mental and overall health of new graduate nurses.[19] As nurses initially enter the practice setting, or change their practice specialty, they lack confidence and may be fearful of making errors.[20] Compounding this fear is the reality of workplace incivility resulting in nurses feeling overwhelmed, ultimately impacting the quality of patient care.[21,22]

Training, including preceptorship and clinical supervision, has been shown to be effective in fostering nurse retention.[23] Preceptors, more experienced and "seasoned" registered nurses, influence the integration experience of nurses during initial or specialty practice orientation; yet research has shown that nurse preceptors frequently feel ill-equipped for this responsibility.[24] Burnout may actually have a negative effect on the relationship between preceptor and preceptee, resulting in transfer of negative attitudes from the preceptor to the orienting nurse.[25] Although research on nurse burnout has focused on detailing nurses' experiences, less emphasis has been placed on understanding relationships and role transition interventions.[26] Strategies that foster nurse integration, such as residency programs and preceptorships, have shown potential in improving retention rates with research revealing the 1-year retention rates for nurses engaged in these programs as high as 90%.[27] Organizations that have a new graduate nurse transition program can ease the stressful shift from student to the reality of becoming a practicing nurse with all of the responsibilities the role entails.[28] Innovative recruitment, onboarding, and burnout prevention interventions for all nursing staff represent potential solutions.

Strategies to Reduce Nurse Burnout

The importance of preceptors: from novice to expert and back

Preceptorship is used by health care organizations to onboard nurses as they acclimate to the health care setting, including assisting with the transition from academia to actual patient care. Although preceptor-preceptee relationships are often discussed in the setting of new graduate nurses, precepted experiences also occur as a nurse transitions to a new clinical area or specialty. Nurse preceptors are required to be competent and current in clinical practice, professional, and objective in providing feedback and to understand the nursing role.[29] Preceptors are often expected to take on this responsibility without receiving adequate training.[30] Precepting requires additional time, energy, and added expectations of carrying out patient duties and explaining procedures to preceptees. Numerous challenges, including stress owing to time constraints and heavy clinical workload, have been reported by preceptors.[31,32] These time constraints may hinder proper acquisition of essential skills, which are key to fostering a positive teaching-learning environment, for both the preceptor and the preceptee.[31] Time constraints also affect relationship building, as preceptors may struggle to find sufficient time for their preceptees.[33]

Research has shown that nurse preceptors may feel inadequately supported by organizational leadership, causing them to have a perception of vulnerability.[29] Preceptors require adequate evidence-based preparation to effectively guide and educate nurses.[34] Time management strategies, ways to foster critical thinking based on adult learning principles, and provision of constructive, professional feedback are among the essential components of preceptor training.[35] When health care organizations fail to provide adequate support and time considerations for preceptors, the preceptee may be viewed as a burden, weakening the preceptor-preceptee relationship. This can initiate a downward spiral of broken professional nurse alliances, relationships that are vital to individual nurse fulfillment and professional satisfaction.

Clinical teaching behaviors are defined as the verbal and nonverbal communications and actions of preceptors that enable learning outcomes in clinical settings.[30] These behaviors include showing concern and support for colleagues.[36] Although there is little research examining preceptor training and the actual effect of such training on the clinical teaching behaviors, preparation that includes education of preceptors through role-playing likely has a positive influence on clinical training behaviors.[37] Fostering communication strategies through role-playing of "difficult conversations" and patient care scenarios offers a potential path forward toward reducing the stress of interdisciplinary relationships, which contribute to development of burnout.

Nurses' satisfaction and intention to stay in their position following initial onboarding are positively influenced by factors such as having one-to-one support and shared workload.[23] Nurse preceptors benefit from organizational support, such as reduced clinical assignments, smaller number of preceptees, and more frequent opportunity to work with the preceptee.[30] Organizational recognition for preceptor ability and clinical expertise is key to their continued commitment.[38] Although the acute care setting offers opportunity to onboard and mentor new nurses, ensuring that outpatient nurses have adequate precepting opportunities is essential to keeping non–hospital-based nurses engaged.[29] The exact role and definition of preceptorship require further study.[39]

Nurse residencies: reducing burnout begins at the start

The American Academy of Nursing (AAN) recommends a residency program for all new graduate nurses.[40] Structured transition to practice programs and residencies can improve safety practices, increase professional satisfaction, and decrease nurse turnover.[41] There is evidence that nurse residencies are not an option but necessary to ensure successful transition to practice, satisfaction, and subsequent retention.[42] Although the ideal length of residency varies, transition to practice programs continuing from 27 to 52 weeks, combining formal instruction and preceptorship, appear to reduce nurse burnout.[43] Organizational networking, including both leadership and staff, with those who have successfully implemented accredited, evidence-based residency programs offers the opportunities for shared standards on how to operationalize the recommendations offered by the AAN.[44] Structured nurse transition to practice programs that incorporate the following appear to provide higher level of support:

> [P]atient-centered care, quality improvement, evidence-based practice, communication and teamwork, informatics, safety, clinical reasoning, feedback, reflection, and knowledge related to the specialty area.[45]

The Commission on Collegiate Nursing Education (CCNE) proposes a nurse residency as a sequence of didactic and clinical learning experiences over a 12-month period to assist new graduates in transitioning to their first professional nursing role.[46] These residencies are offered collaboratively between academic nursing programs and health care organizations. The American Nurse Credentialing Center (ANCC) defines a nurse residency as an evidence-based program, of at least 6-months' duration, by which licensed registered nurses with less than 12 months of experience can develop the knowledge, clinical skills, and professional behaviors essential to delivery of quality care, including orientation to the health care organization and practice-based experience.[47] Nurses who participated in a 12-month residency program have reported a significant increase in their ability to prioritize work with increased comfort in communicating with health care team members and patients.[40]

Key elements of transition programs include clinical coaching by a preceptor, simulation, and participation in committees[10] with a principal goal being provision of support to nurses as they develop applicable clinical skills. Although safety is a primary objective of a successful transition, coaching for the development of communication skills, offering strategies to deal with workplace incivility, teamwork, and definition of the professional nurse role are equally essential components of a residency program.[48] Nurse residency-transition programs can significantly reduce turnover and burnout and can also positively impact nurse competencies, job satisfaction, self-confidence, and group cohesion.[49] There are reports that organizations may yield a financial benefit when implementing a transition program, likely because of higher retention rates.[50]

The Magnet Recognition Program has been identified as having elements of support for professional nurses, which improves working conditions and, as an outcome, reduces their professional attrition and increases patient satisfaction.[51] In an effort to standardize nurse residency programs, the ANCC Practice Transition Accreditation Program (PTAP) accreditation framework has been recognized by more than 100 transition-to-practice programs in the United States and incorporated as a source of evidence in the 2019 Magnet Recognition Program Manual.[52] The ANCC PTAP best practice recommendations include (a) inclusion of a quality improvement data analyst and evaluation measures, (b) need for an off-shift nurse educator, (c) application of evidence-based practice, and (d) a uniform preceptor program. Residency and transition program accreditation continues to evolve; therefore, resources related to the actual application process are limited. Although standardized guidelines continue to develop, involvement of organization administration, nurse leaders, and direct care nurses in the accreditation process is central to success. Consistency across programs will be essential to ensure they are evidence-based and support accreditation.[44]

Journal clubs can be incorporated into residencies or unit-based council meetings and have been found to be helpful for nurses, as a way to meet with colleagues in a more social sense.[52] Beck and colleagues[53] proposed that human learning is a lifelong process; a journal club can be a good supplement to formal training and practice education. These researchers propose that learning through reflection and collaborative discussion can foster trust and valuing of evidence-based practice. Discussion shared among colleagues can help to narrate practice experiences and form professional interdisciplinary team identity. The sense of being a part of a team can help prevent burnout during prolonged stress.

Critical thinking and clinical reasoning can be promoted through use of case studies and reflection. Evidence shows that nurses without adequate clinical reasoning training and skill development may fail to identify the subtle early signs of clinical deterioration placing patients at increased safety risk.[54] Created simulations incorporated within the structure of a transition program can increase nurses' critical thinking skills and foster confidence, which are essential to addressing burnout, especially in early career nurses.

Although nurse transition programs may reduce burnout and turnover,[49] there is a need to continue to evaluate the actual experience of all nurses to identify specific, standard strategies that can facilitate successful professional integration and identity. The key is providing a concentrated clinical experience that approximates professional practice expectations.[55,56]

Clinical Relevance of Burnout

"Do I have it or am I just having a bad day?"

It is crucial for all nurses to know the signs and symptoms of burnout and possible behaviors exhibited in the workplace. Frequently, behaviors present in the workplace setting include but are not limited to the following[57]:

- Loss of tolerance when attending to patient care

- Medication and treatment errors
- Irritability with peers
- Absence from unit with no notification to peers or manager
- Exchanges with patients, peers, or superiors that are brief and lack sufficient details
- Lack of support of organization's initiatives or policies

Knowing the behavior clues can help to identify signs and symptoms of burnout. These may be displayed in the clinical setting or in the nurse's personal life[58]:

- Insomnia/hypersomnia
- Weight loss or weight gain
- Irritability with family
- Argumentative
- Decreased libido
- Increased self-doubt
- Lack of self-discipline
- Crying easily with limited provocation
- Exhibiting self-destructive behavior

What can I do if I feel "burnt-out"?

Daily sustained self-care and becoming *self-directed* as opposed to *other-directed* are key. There are simple mechanisms for relieving burnout,[59,60] as follows:

- The best intervention is prevention
  - Getting proper rest
  - Balanced diet
  - Time for yourself with no interruptions
  - Talk to your nurse leader, or manager, about distress you may be feeling and try to negotiate for improved working conditions, for example, change in hours, personal time off, and so forth
  - Discuss working conditions during shared governance or unit-based meetings
  - Incorporate mindfulness activities, for example, including yoga, meditation, and guided imagery
  - Maintain a personalized, consistent exercise regimen
  - Balance work and relaxation: Be sure to plan activities you enjoy with people you enjoy spending time with
  - Set goals and objectives for your life
  - Seek and take advantage of continuing education, both formal and informal
  - Take scheduled breaks and lunch periods; avoid discussing work with your peers at these times

Developing resilience

The concept of resilience has several common elements. Essentially, resilience is a state of recovery, or a return to a previous state after a time of stress or adverse event.[61] Protective factors that foster resilience have been proposed and can be described as follows:

- *Positive emotions*: Trying to see the positive in situations, even if they are disappointing, and learning from them, avoiding gossip and complaining, being supportive of others
- *Being hopeful*: Believing that something better is possible
- *Optimism*: Trying to see the best in every situation

- *Perseverance*: Believing that you can overcome barriers and achieve your goals, even when faced with adversity
- *Being self-aware*: Recognizing your strengths as well as your limitations, focus on personal priorities even during stressful times, know your worth
- *Stay adaptable*: Trying cooperation, being more tolerant, responding positively when asked to make a change
- *Do not underestimate your social support system*: Staying close to family and friends, especially those who bring you joy and unconditional love; distance yourself from negative people and avoid their influence

Having a personal reflective journal can be helpful. Although the journal is personal, it can be used to self-reflect on concerns or stressors when they occur and later can be shared with trusted others as feels comfortable.[62]

A word about gratitude
Gratitude is a vaccine, an antitoxin, and an antiseptic.
— John Henry Jowett, 1863–1923

Gratitude can motivate people to make positive changes in their lives and in the world around them.[63] Embracing feelings of connectedness, humility, and generosity can enhance psychological and physical well-being and may actually alter biomarkers that predict risk for cardiovascular disease.[64]

- *Connectedness*: Gratitude rewards us with a strong network of support and encouragement, leading us feel we can take on challenges
- *Elevation*: Gratitude inspires and motivates us to become healthier, more generous and productive workers
- *Humility*: Expressing gratitude highlights how other people have contributed to the successes in our lives
- *Generosity*: Gratitude encourages us to recognize, reward, and "pay forward" the good others have offered us, reinforcing the gratification of kindness

Research has demonstrated that positive emotions, including gratitude, are analogous to health and wellness. Being grateful is a mindfulness practice to help cope with stress and uncertainty, shifting focus to those things and people that are valuable in our lives, what we can control, and what we can give back.[65]

Being present in the moment during caregiving activities and appreciating the experience offer an opportunity for gratitude reflection. Take a few deep breaths and allow yourself to be thankful for the healing nursing profession of which you have the honor of being part.[63]

What can organizations do?
Mindfulness has been defined as the "practice of learning to focus attention and awareness on the moment-by-moment experience with an attitude of curiosity, openness and acceptance."[66] Mindfulness and resilience training provided by organizations can increase nurse retention and reduce turnover.[67] These strategies alone do not adequately address burnout; however, when incorporated with supportive leadership behaviors that empower nurses, they can be helpful, even in reducing medication errors and safety events.

Leadership is complex,[68] occurring in formal, appointed positions or in informal roles that nurses assume.

Let whoever is in charge keep this simple question in her head (not, how can I always do this right thing myself, but) how can I provide for this right thing to be always done?

Florence Nightingale, 1860

Empowering leadership behaviors include giving employees the ability to access resources and support needed to perform their work. Several factors can be engaged by leaders to support nurses in their professional nursing roles, as follows[66]:

- Promote opportunities for nursing participation in decision making
- Give staff a chance to voice opinions related to their work
- *Build* confidence by *expressing* confidence in the ability of each nurse to meet and exceed expectations
- Recognize and reward accomplishments
- Freely share resources and opportunities

Organizational leaders must create a culture of ethical practice offering nurses education and mentoring to develop relational skills, such as introspection, empathy, communication, and mindfulness. The practice environment should foster professional communication and reward nurses for raising ethical questions. Nursing ethics "huddles" may be considered when ethically challenging issues occur.[69] Provide support for nurses as they question and apply evidence-based nursing science principles. Inspire and coach nurses to comfortably initiate PRN ("as-needed") discussions with physicians or other relevant health care colleagues.

Future Directions

Compassion satisfaction: accentuate the positive

Compassion satisfaction is defined as the pleasure of your professional work and positivity about professional relationships, including having a sense of contributing to the greater good of society through working with those who need care and the experience of fulfillment resulting from the work of caring for others.[70] Compassion satisfaction is a positive approach to preventing burnout and affects the quality of nursing care, which is predictive of patient satisfaction.[71] Research has suggested that collegial professional relationships among providers are protective against the negative aspects of workload and demands of clinical care, resulting in lower levels of burnout and higher compassion satisfaction.[72] There is evidence of the relationship between self-care strategies and reduced burnout and association with higher levels of compassion satisfaction with compassion satisfaction.[73]

There is a paucity of research related to the prevalence and predictors of compassion satisfaction in nurses and other health care providers. Interestingly, pediatric palliative care providers report high levels of compassion satisfaction, finding their work rewarding despite the challenges of providing comfort rather than curative care to children.[74] Future research is warranted evaluating "connecting to purpose" as a result of providing nursing care and the effect on compassion, perspective, and burnout.

CASE STUDY: A NURSE IN THE EMERGENCY DEPARTMENT
Case Review

Jennifer is a 39-year-old, white woman who graduated with her BSN degree from the local university 3 years ago. After spending her initial 2 years of practice in the medical-surgical unit of the hospital, she was recently transferred to the Emergency Department (ED), fulfilling her dream of emergency service practice. She was assigned a preceptor in the ED for several weeks, and although she initially felt ill-prepared to take on the independent ED nurse role, she felt that she could work independently with a "shadow" preceptor for support. After being in the ED for approximately 6 months, she found herself experiencing headaches, feeling very tired in the morning, with difficulty getting out of bed and going to work. What she discovered was that the schedule that she was initially assigned was not being kept and that her schedule was being modified almost every 2 weeks. Her ED preceptor was now assigned to another shift and was no longer available. It was becoming increasingly difficult for her to plan any family activities because of the disrupted work schedule. She went to her supervisor to discuss this issue, and the supervisor indicated that there was nothing she could do to rectify the situation, leaving Jennifer feeling very much unheard. The nurse started taking longer lunch periods and often was difficult to locate, which led her to a write-up and formal performance warning from her manager for a "poor work ethic." At home, she found herself frustrated with her children and often in arguments with her spouse over various issues. She only looked forward to her days off, but they were filled with so many tasks to complete that she was feeling as if she never had any time for herself. She often dreamed of being able to quit her job and becoming a stay-at-home mom; however, finances could not be managed as a one-income family. She felt very frustrated and bewildered and was very disappointed with her life. She frequently questions nursing as a meaningful, "making-a-difference" profession.

Case Questions to Consider

1. How might you encourage time management strategies? What would these specific strategies be?
2. Is it OK to say no? When and how would you support this nurse to avoid taking on more than she can handle and to set limits?
3. What self-care practices would you suggest?
4. Would you advise her to speak with her supervisor, coworker, friend? Who, why, or why not?
5. Does she need professional help? Is there a mechanism for her to request a referral (or be referred) to a counseling professional, human resources, or employee assistance?
6. How would you let her know she is not alone?

SUMMARY

Nurse burnout is a concern that is real, for the nursing profession, individual nurses, and health care organizations. Patient safety concerns, staffing, bullying, poor communication with colleagues, and workplace incivility can contribute to nurse burnout and dissatisfaction, often influencing a nurse's decision to leave their first position and, in some cases, the profession.

It is important to appreciate that nurse burnout will not go away on its own and does require active intervention. New graduate nurses are at increased risk for early career burnout; however, as nurses are increasingly being asked to move from novice to expert and back, as demonstrated in the COVID-19 pandemic, all nurses are at burnout risk. Nurses are being asked to apply rapidly evolving evidence to practice, cope with ongoing stress, and self-renew when exhausted. It is vital that nurses find balance between professional activity and personal time away from work, where they have opportunities to do things for themselves and their family, giving a sense of a holistic life.

Providing support, training, and professional development opportunities to nurses identified as preceptors is imperative. Nursing leadership needs to role model positive actions and strategies, offering reward, recognition, and reinforcement to novice and experienced nurses, such as preceptors. Nurses' irreplaceable contribution to the organization and patient care quality must be freely spoken and hardwired within the organizational mission. Individual and organizational interventions to increase a nurse's protective factors should be emphasized and encouraged, targeted to those protective factors that the individual nurse has identified. Mindfulness and development of resilience strategies have been identified as positive influences in reducing burnout turnover and deserve further study.

Although more research is needed to develop and standardize the role of nurse residency and transition programs, organization investment in such programs offers a potential strategy to address the critical nature of nurse retention while fostering nurse preceptor training. Standardization of nurse residencies and transition programs leading to accreditation likely offer a pathway to further research and measurement of such programs in reducing nurse burnout and attrition.

An important area for future research is the use of role-play in preceptor-preceptee training to foster clinical teaching of interprofessional communication, including nurse-physician dialogue. Role-playing that portrays difficult conversations and stressful circumstances offers an opportunity to enhance professional communication skills within a safe, realistic clinical setting, leveraging peers and preceptors. Effective communication across organizations and disciplines, including active listening and feedback of what is heard, is an effective strategy in reducing nurse burnout and turnover. Future research on the actual effect of role-playing in the early career experience of nurses and subsequent retention is needed and warranted.

High levels of compassion satisfaction appears to have an inverse relationship with burnout. Specific predictors of compassion satisfaction in nurses and other health care providers, such as practice specialty and perception of belonging to a team who together are dedicated to patient outcomes, are important to future interdisciplinary research. Connecting to a purpose that emanates from the heart as a result of inner reflection and introspection following challenging clinical experiences may be what shifts a nurse from the brink of irrevocable burnout to motivation and engagement. It is a fertile area for research, evaluating strategies to reduce nurse burnout.

Nothing truly valuable arises from ambition or from a mere sense of duty; it stems rather from love and devotion towards men and towards objective things.
—*Albert Einstein*

DISCLOSURE

The authors have nothing to disclose.

REFERENCES

1. Maslach C, Schaufeli WB, Leiter MP. Job burnout. Annu Rev Psychol 2001;52: 397–422.

2. World Health Organization. Burn-out an "occupational phenomenon": International Classification of Diseases. 2019. Available at: https://www.who.int/news/item/28-05-2019-burn-out-an-occupational-phenomenon-international-classification-of-diseases. Accessed June 15, 2021.

3. Reith TP. Burnout in United States healthcare professionals: a narrative review. Cureus 2018;10(12):e3681.

4. Rushton CH, Batcheller J, Schroeder K, et al. Burnout and resilience among nurses practicing in high-intensity settings. Am J Crit Care 2015;24(5):412-20.

5. Laschinger HK, Wong CA, Grau AL. Authentic leadership, empowerment and burnout: a comparison in new graduates and experienced nurses. J Nurs Manag 2013;21(3):541-52.

6. Kim JS. Emotional labor strategies, stress, and burnout among hospital nurses: a path analysis. J Nurs Scholarsh 2020;52(1):105-12.

7. Sharma J, Dhar RL. Factors influencing job performance of nursing staff: mediating role of affective commitment. Personnel Rev 2016;45(1).

8. Gardiner I, Sheen J. Graduate nurse experiences of support: a review. Nurse Education Today 2016;40:7-12.

9. Phillips C, Kenny A, Esterman A. Supporting graduate nurse transition to practice through a quality assurance feedback loop. Nurse Education Pract 2017;27: 121-7.

10. Twibell R, Pierre J St, Johnson D, et al. Why new nurses don't stay and what the evidence says we can do about it. Am Nurse Today 2012;7(6).

11. Ray-Sannerud BN, Leyshon S, Vallevik VB. Introducing routine measurement of healthcare worker's well-being as a leading indicator for proactive safety management systems based on resilience engineering. Proced Manufacturing 2015;3:319-26.

12. Shah MK, Gandrakota N, Cimiotti JP, et al. Prevalence of and factors associated with nurse burnout in the US. JAMA Netw open 2021;4(2):e2036469.

13. Rhéaume A, Clément L, Lebel N. Understanding intention to leave amongst new graduate Canadian nurses: a repeated cross sectional survey. Int J Nurs Stud 2011;48(4):490-500.

14. Laschinger HK, Grau AL. The influence of personal dispositional factors and organizational resources on workplace violence, burnout, and health outcomes in new graduate nurses: a cross-sectional study. Int J Nurs Stud 2012;49(3): 282-91.

15. Parker V, Giles M, Lantry G, et al. New graduate nurses' experiences in their first year of practice. Nurse Education Today 2014;34(1):150-6.

16. Ahola K, Kivimäki M, Honkonen T, et al. Occupational burnout and medically certified sickness absence: a population-based study of Finnish employees. J Psychosomatic Res 2008;64(2):185-93.

17. Smiley RA, Ruttinger C, Oliveira CM, et al. The 2020 National Nursing Workforce Survey. J Nurs Regul 2021;12(1):S4-96.

18. Sandler M. Why are new graduate nurses leaving the profession in their first year of practice and how does this impact on ED nurse staffing? A rapid review of current literature and recommended reading. CJEN 2020;41(1):23-4. Available at: https://cjen.ca/index.php/cjen/article/view/66. Accessed July10, 2021.

19. Johnson SL, Rea RE. Workplace bullying: concerns for nurse leaders. J Nurs Adm 2009;39(2):84-90.

20. Wing T, Regan S, Spence Laschinger HK. The influence of empowerment and incivility on the mental health of new graduate nurses. J Nurs Management 2015;23(5):632-43.

21. Laschinger HK, Wong C, Regan S, et al. Workplace incivility and new graduate nurses' mental health: the protective role of resiliency. J Nurs Adm 2013; 43(7/8):415-21.

22. Laschinger HK. Impact of workplace mistreatment on patient safety risk and nurse-assessed patient outcomes. J Nurs Adm 2014;44(5):284–90.
23. Aparício C, Nicholson J. Do preceptorship and clinical supervision programmes support the retention of nurses? Br J Nurs 2020;29(20):1192–7.
24. Edward KL, Ousey K, Playle J, et al. Are new nurses work ready–the impact of preceptorship. An integrative systematic review. J Prof Nurs 2017;33(5):326–33.
25. Frankenberger WD, Roberts KE, Hutchins L, et al. Experience of burnout among pediatric inpatient nurse preceptors. Nurse Education Today 2021;100:104862.
26. Kenny A, Dickson-Swift V, McKenna L, et al. Interventions to support graduate nurse transition to practice and associated outcomes: a systematic review. Nurse Education Today 2021;104860.
27. Spence Laschinger HK, Wong C, Read E, et al. Predictors of new graduate nurses' health over the first 4 years of practice. Nurs Open 2018;6(2):245–59.
28. Rush KL, Janke R, Duchscher JE, et al. Best practices of formal new graduate transition programs: an integrative review. Int J Nurs Stud 2019;94:139–58.
29. Ong SL, Ang WHD, Goh LJ, et al. Understanding nurse preceptors' experiences in a primary health care setting: a descriptive qualitative study. J Nurs Manag 2021;29(5):1320–8. https://doi.org/10.1111/jonm.13272.
30. Hong KJ, Yoon HJ. Effect of nurses' preceptorship experience in educating new graduate nurses and preceptor training courses on clinical teaching behavior. Int J Environ Res Public Health 2021;18(3):975.
31. Chan HY, So WK, Aboo G, et al. Understanding the needs of nurse preceptors in acute hospital care setting: a mixed-method study. Nurse Education Pract 2019; 38:112–9.
32. Tracey JM, McGowan IW. Preceptors' views on their role in supporting newly qualified nurses. Br J Nurs 2015;24(20):998–1001.
33. Staples E, Sangster-Gormley E. Supporting nurse practitioner education: preceptorship recruitment and retention. Int J Nurs Sci 2018;5(2):115–20.
34. Cadmus E, Salmond SW, Hassler LJ, et al. Creating a long-term care new nurse residency model. J Continuing Education Nurs 2016;47(5):234–40.
35. Bohnarczyk N, Cadmus E. Preceptor criteria revisited. The J Continuing Education Nurs 2020;51(9):425–32.
36. Lee-Hsieh J, O'Brien A, Liu CY, et al. The development and validation of the Clinical Teaching Behavior Inventory (CTBI-23): nurse preceptors' and new graduate nurses' perceptions of precepting. Nurse Education Today 2016;38:107–14.
37. Rønning SB, Bjørkly S. The use of clinical role-play and reflection in learning therapeutic communication skills in mental health education: an integrative review. Adv Med Education Pract 2019;10:415.
38. Chen F, Liu Y, Wang X, et al. Transition shock, preceptor support and nursing competency among newly graduated registered nurses: a cross-sectional study. Nurse Education Today 2021;102:104891.
39. Irwin C, Bliss J, Poole K. Does preceptorship improve confidence and competence in newly qualified nurses: a systematic literature review. Nurse Education Today 2018;60:35–46.
40. Goode CJ, Glassman KS, Ponte PR, et al. Requiring a nurse residency for newly licensed registered nurses. Nurs Outlook 2018;66(3):329–32.
41. Kramer M, Maguire P, Halfer D, et al. The organizational transformative power of nurse residency programs. Nurs Adm Q 2012;36(2):155–68.
42. Lin PS, Viscardi MK, McHugh MD. Factors influencing job satisfaction of new graduate nurses participating in nurse residency programs: a systematic review. J Continuing Education Nurs 2014;45(10):439–50.

43. Brook J, Aitken LM, MacLaren JA, et al. An intervention to decrease burnout and increase retention of early career nurses: a mixed methods study of acceptability and feasibility. BMC Nurs 2021;20(1):1–2.

44. Trepanier S, Yoder-Wise PS, Church CD, et al. Nurse leaders' assumptions and attitudes toward residency programs for new graduate nurses. Nurs Adm Q 2021;45(1):26–34.

45. Spector N, Blegen MA, Silvestre J, et al. Transition to practice study in hospital settings. J Nurs Regul 2015;5(4):24–38.

46. Commission on Collegiate Nursing Education. Standards for accreditation of entry-to-practice nurse residency programs 2021. Available at: https://www.aacnnursing.org/Portals/42/CCNE/PDF/CCNE-Entry-to-Practice-Residency-Standards-2021.pdf. Accessed June 15, 2021.

47. American Nurses Credentialling Center. Practice Transition Accreditation Program® (PTAP). Available at: https://www.nursingworld.org/organizational-programs/accreditation/ptap/. Accessed June 15, 2021.

48. Clark CM, Springer PJ. Nurse residents' first-hand accounts on transition to practice. Nurs Outlook 2012;60(4):e2–8.

49. Pittman P, Herrera C, Bass E, et al. Residency programs for new nurse graduates: how widespread are they and what are the primary obstacles to further adoption? J Nurs Adm 2013;43(11):597–602.

50. Ackerson K, Stiles KA. Value of nurse residency programs in retaining new graduate nurses and their potential effect on the nursing shortage. J Contin Educ Nurs 2018;49(6):282–8.

51. Schlak AE, Aiken LH, Chittams J, et al. Leveraging the work environment to minimize the negative impact of nurse burnout on patient outcomes. Int J Environ Res Public Health 2021;18(2):610.

52. Church CD, Cosme S, O'Brien M. Accreditation of transition to practice programs: assessing the value and impact. J Nurses Prof Development 2019; 35(4):180–4.

53. Beck M, Simonÿ C, Bergenholtz H, et al. Professional consciousness and pride facilitate evidence-based practice—the meaning of participating in a journal club based on clinical practice reflection. Nurs Open 2020;7(3):690–9.

54. Lapkin S, Levett-Jones T, Bellchambers H, et al. Effectiveness of patient simulation manikins in teaching clinical reasoning skills to undergraduate nursing students: a systematic review. Clin Simulation Nurs 2010;6(6):e207–22.

55. Fowler SM, Knowlton MC, Putnam AW. Reforming the undergraduate nursing clinical curriculum through clinical immersion: a literature review. Nurse Education Pract 2018;31:68–76.

56. Tratnack SA, O'Neill CM, Graham P. Immersion experience in undergraduate psychiatric mental health nursing. J Nurs Education 2011;50(9):532–5.

57. Brown LW, Quick JC. Environmental influences on individual burnout and a preventive approach for organizations. J Appl Biobehavioral Res 2013;18(2):104–21.

58. Mayo Clinic. Job burnout: how to spot it and take action 2021. Available at: https://www.mayoclinic.org/healthy-lifestyle/adult-health/in-depth/burnout/art-20046642. Accessed June 15, 2021.

59. Pruthi NR, Deal A, Langston J, et al. Factors related to job satisfaction in urology. Urol Pract 2016 May;3(3):169–74.

60. Brandsma R. The mindfulness teaching guide: essential skills and competencies for teaching mindfulness-based interventions. United States: New Harbinger Publications; 2017.

61. Stephens TM. Nursing student resilience: a concept clarification. Nurs Forum 2013;48(2):125–33.
62. Stevens D, Cooper J. Journal keeping: how to use reflective writing for effective learning, teaching, professional insight, and positive change. Sterling, VA: Stylus Publications. WorldCat; 2009. Available at: http://mcgill.worldcat.org/oclc/646821096.
63. American Nurses Foundation. The Greater Good Science Center at the University of California, Berkeley. Gratitude practice for nurses. Supporting well-being and building a culture of gratitude in nursing. 2021. Available at: https://ggsc.berkeley.edu/gratitudefornurses. Accessed June 15, 2021.
64. Cousin L, Redwine L, Bricker C, et al. Effect of gratitude on cardiovascular health outcomes: a state-of-the-science review. J Positive Psychol 2021;16(3):348–55.
65. Fishman MD. The silver linings journal: gratitude during a pandemic. J Radiol Nurs 2020;39(3):149.
66. The Joint Commission. Quick safety, issue 50: "developing resilience to combat nurse burnout.". 2019. Available at: https://www.jointcommission.org/-/media/tjc/newsletters/quick_safety_nurse_resilience_final_7_19_19pdf.pdf. Accessed June 15, 2021.
67. Magtibay DL, Chesak SS, Coughlin K, et al. Decreasing stress and burnout in nurses: efficacy of blended learning with stress management and resilience training program. J Nurs Adm 2017;47(7/8):391–5.
68. Larsson IE, Sahlsten MJ. The staff nurse clinical leader at the bedside: Swedish registered nurses' perceptions. Nurs Res Pract 2016;2016.
69. Lizarondo L. Evidence summary. Moral distress (nurses): strategies in emergency department settings. The Joanna Briggs Institute EBP Database, JBI@Ovid. 2020; JBI23873
70. Stamm, B.H. The ProQOL (professional quality of life scale: compassion satisfaction and compassion fatigue). Whitefish, MT: ProQOL.org; 2010. Available at: www.proqol.org. Accessed June 15, 2021.
71. Baek J, Cho H, Han K, et al. Association between nursing work environment and compassion satisfaction among clinical nurses. J Nurs Manag 2020;28(2):368–76.
72. Kase SM, Waldman ED, Weintraub AS. A cross-sectional pilot study of compassion fatigue, burnout, and compassion satisfaction in pediatric palliative care providers in the United States. Palliat Support Care 2019;17(3):269–75.
73. Zhang YY, Zhang C, Han XR, et al. Determinants of compassion satisfaction, compassion fatigue and burn out in nursing: a correlative meta-analysis. Medicine (Baltimore) 2018;97(26):e11086.
74. Beaune L, Muskat B, Anthony SJ. The emergence of personal growth amongst healthcare professionals who care for dying children. Palliat Support Care 2018;16(3):298–307.

The Effect of Burnout on Quality of Care Using Donabedian's Framework

Kathleen M. White, PhD, RN, NEA-BC[a],*,
Dorothy Dulko, PhD, ARNP-BC, AOCNP, WHNP-BC[b,1],
Bonnie DiPietro, MS, RN, NEA-BC[c]

KEYWORDS

- Burnout • Quality • Safety • Donabedian • Structure • Process • Outcomes

KEY POINTS

- Burnout has reached concerning levels among health care professionals and can have a negative association with quality and safety outcomes.
- Nurses and physicians are reporting increasing and higher levels of burnout in the workplace.
- The Donabedian model of quality has been applied for decades to frame the interrelationship between health care organization structures, processes, and outcomes of care.
- Attention must be paid to identifying opportunities to implement traditional and innovative organizational strategies to decrease levels of burnout in health care professionals.

INTRODUCTION

Burnout is a syndrome described along the following 3 dimensions: (a) feelings of energy depletion or *emotional exhaustion*; (b) increased mental distance from one's job or *depersonalization*; and (c) reduced professional efficacy or decreased sense of *personal accomplishment*.[1,2] Burnout has reached concerning levels among US health care professionals, with 43% of physicians reporting burnout in 2020, similar to 46% reporting burnout in 2015 and 39.8% reporting burnout in 2013.[3] Nurses report a similarly high percentage of burnout.[4] A second survey was conducted by Berxi, a division of Berkshire Hathaway Specialty Insurance, to learn more about health care workers mental and physical well-being compared with this time last year. Their

[a] Johns Hopkins School of Nursing, 2850 Pebble Beach Drive, Ellicott City, MD 21042, USA; [b] American Association of Colleges of Nursing, 655 K Street, NW, Suite 750, Washington, DC 20001, USA; [c] Maryland Patient Safety Center, 6820 Deerpath Road, Elkridge, MD 21075, USA
[1] The views, analyses, and conclusions expressed in this article are those of the authors and do not necessarily reflect the official policy or positions of the American Association of Colleges of Nursing.
* Corresponding author.
E-mail address: kwhite2@jhu.edu

Nurs Clin N Am 57 (2022) 115–130
https://doi.org/10.1016/j.cnur.2021.11.008
0029-6465/22/© 2021 Elsevier Inc. All rights reserved.

results were even more startling, with the current pandemic compounding burnout feelings, with 84% of survey respondents reporting feeling at least mildly burned out from work, and 18% feeling totally burned out. The top 5 stressors they reported were fear of getting COVID-19; long hours/shifts; the general state of the world; fear of spreading the coronavirus; and family issues and responsibilities.[5]

The effects of burnout are not limited to the personal well-being of health care workers; they have implications for employer organizations, patients, and the entire health care system.[6] The increased incidence of health care worker burnout has been associated with rising patient safety incidents, including medical errors, reduced patient satisfaction, and poor safety and quality ratings.[7,8] Although the relationship between health care burnout and quality of care is suggested, research establishing a direct relationship between these 2 constructs has varied across specialties and domains of quality, for example, patient satisfaction, medical and nursing errors, with too few studies conducted to definitively propose a causal relationship.

Avedis Donabedian, a physician and health services researcher at the University of Michigan, defined the 7 attributes of health care quality as efficacy, effectiveness, efficiency, optimality, acceptability, legitimacy, and equity.[9] The Donabedian model of quality has been applied for decades to frame the interrelationship between health care organization structures, processes, and outcomes of care. The model proposes that structure, process, and outcomes are closely linked and determine outcomes.[10] This model, including organizational structure and process workflows, can be applied to evaluate the outcomes of health care quality interventions on health care worker burnout.[11]

Structural measures are described as characteristics of institutions and providers, the space and manner in which health care occurs, including architecture, availability of equipment, and human resources. Process measures include delivery of care to health care clients, the interactions between providers and clients, and the workflows of diagnosis, treatment, prevention, rehabilitation, and education. Outcome measures describe the effects of health care on the health status of clients and populations or what happens to the health care client as a result of health care interactions/interventions resulting in changes in health status, behavior, knowledge, satisfaction, and quality of life.

ASSOCIATION OF BURNOUT FACTORS RELATED TO QUALITY OF CARE: ARE THERE PREDICTORS?

Tawfik and colleagues[12,13] reported a systematic review and meta-analysis that attempted to quantify the relationship between burnout and quality of care over 25 years. The researchers noted that there were few rigorous studies, as most included studies were cross-sectional, observational research that could not determine the directionality of a causal relationship. An interesting question is whether curtailing burnout improves quality of care or whether improving quality of care reduces burnout.

Structure

Use of Donabedian's model in health services is helpful to conceptualize and evaluate quality in health care. Evaluation of structure assists in identifying the presence of the institutional and provider resources necessary to predict a possible association between burnout and quality and safety concerns.

The consequences of burnout among nursing staff have been shown to result in lack of teamwork, decreased job performance, increased workload, lack of control/autonomy, job dissatisfaction, increased absenteeism, and intention to leave.[14–18]

In a cross-sectional study, Lowe and colleagues[19] evaluated structure by studying the relationship among burnout, coworker support, and the nursing practice environment in a national sample of palliative care staff nurses. Burnout was measured using the 9-item Emotional Exhaustion subscale of the Maslach Burnout Inventory (MBI). More than 70% of palliative care nurses studied reported experiencing moderate to high burnout. Perception of lack of organizational and coworker support was a strong predictor of burnout in this group of nurses. Salyers and colleagues[6] found that having a consistent role within the health care organization may be an important variable in reducing burnout, with higher nurse-to-patient staffing ratios and perceived poor organizational communication being potential predictors of burnout.

Binder and colleagues[11] reported the results of a quality improvement (QI) project implemented in a 292-bed nonprofit medical center during the COVID-19 pandemic. Using Donabedian's quality framework, the QI team evaluated emergency department (ED) structure measures, including physical design, to prepare for ongoing and future infectious disease crises and potential natural disasters. The QI interventions included triage addition of a "quick-look" waiting room registered nurse (RN), addressing staff morale and use of telehealth. Creating a permanent ED waiting room RN was reported as a key structural improvement measure, particularly in early identification of infection control risks to hospital staff and patients. The use of telehealth was seen as helpful in triaging patients and minimizing direct infection exposure to patients and staff. As care processes were continually changing, staff members reported feeling uninformed as they arrived for their shift each day. Hospital leadership responded to this concern by implementing a daily briefing that included a summary of changes in patient and staff safety measures that had occurred in the prior 24 hours. A staff online portal was created whereby most current processes and procedures were posted. This online portal also served as a staff blog, allowing secure Web-based interstaff discussions in real time. Positive feedback related to communication was noted. They noted that further study postpandemic is needed to confirm the effect of continued Web-based policy, procedures, and safety measures.

Spence Laschinger and Leiter[20] tested a theoretic model linking the professional nursing environment to an association with burnout. They found that nursing leadership played an important role in the quality of work life and that adequate staffing directly affected emotional exhaustion (burnout dimension) and patient safety outcomes. Liu and Aungsuroch[21] also developed and tested a theoretic model from a cross-sectional survey that evaluated work environment, patient-to-nurse ratio, job satisfaction, burnout, intention to leave, and quality care with nurses in China. The proposed model was supported with work environment having a large total effect size on quality nursing care and burnout affecting and directly influencing quality nursing care, which was followed by work environment and patient-to-nurse ratio.

The literature includes studies that found structural factors, such as ineffective teamwork, failed organizational process, loss of control or autonomy, and the physical and psychological overload of health professionals, are known to compromise patient safety and are also associated with burnout.[22,23] Alves and colleagues[24] found nurses with greater autonomy, good working relationships, and control over their environment have lower levels of emotional exhaustion. Profit and colleagues[25] reported that neonatal intensive care units (ICUs) with higher burnout scores had a lower teamwork climate, safety climate, job satisfaction, and lower perceptions of management and working conditions. Likewise, Van Bogaert and colleagues[26] studied the nurse practice environment and nurse work characteristics and found unit-level associations to burnout and reported quality measures. Finally, Guirardello[27] reported that professionals who perceived greater autonomy, good relationships with the medical team, and better control over the work environment also presented lower levels of burnout and reported a positive perception on safety attitude for the job satisfaction domain.

Researchers at the Mayo Clinic have been studying burnout among physicians for almost 10 years. In 2015, they found that 40% of physicians reported at least 1 symptom of burnout, and that burnout rates were higher in physicians who rated their leaders unfavorably. They also found that, even in a physician group with high satisfaction ratings (79% satisfied or very satisfied), leadership quality explained almost half the variation in physician satisfaction scores. This study highlights the importance of organizational leadership to clinician well-being.[28] Another important study in 2015 involved a randomized controlled trial that measured the impact of changes in work conditions on clinician stress and burnout.[29] These investigators collected baseline assessments of clinician burnout, working conditions, and quality metrics in 166 physicians, nurse practitioners, and physician assistants in 34 primary care clinics. The clinics were then divided into intervention and control groups. The clinicians in the intervention practices selected from a list of options for improvement focused on enhancing communication, clinician workflow, or another area that might influence a clinician-selected quality metric. Once selected, the entire clinic adopted the intervention. The study's results were promising. The intervention clinics that focused on workflow improvements or targeted QI projects saw significantly reduced rates of burnout. The intervention clinics that chose to address improvements in communication saw increased rates of clinician satisfaction. These results support the idea that the odds of achieving the so-called Triple Aim (improving the patient experience of care, improving the health of the population, and reducing per-capita costs) are markedly enhanced when clinicians are satisfied. However, over the last 5 years, the health care work environment has continued to undergo fast-paced changes leading to increased provider stress and burnout. In a recent editorial, Sikka and colleagues[30] supported Bodenheimer and Sinsky's premise that clinician well-being is foundational to achieving the goals of the Triple Aim and should be renamed the Quadruple Aim to include provider well-being or achieving meaning or accomplishment in work.[31,32]

Process

The identification and evaluation of process measures are critical to the understanding of key interactions between providers and clients that can predict a possible association between burnout and quality and safety concerns. Park and Hwang[33] analyzed questionnaires from more than 300 nurses working in 7 small and medium-sized general hospitals. Nonnursing tasks and nursing care left undone were associated with nurse burnout, intent to leave nursing positions, and an increased incidence of medical errors.

In a cross-sectional, exploratory study, Liu and colleagues[34] measured organizational factors, such as workload, with processes being defined as nursing care left undone, and outcomes, including nurse burnout, specifically emotional exhaustion. They found that lower dayshift patient-nurse ratios correlated with fewer nursing care tasks left undone, less burnout, and improved nurse perceptions of patient safety. Patient safety was evaluated using 3 items assessing nurses' perception of patient safety and 9 items addressing patient adverse events. The researchers reported that providing support for nurses and enabling more time for direct patient care activities may help to reduce burnout and promote patient safety.

A hospital medicine leadership team at the University of Colorado surveyed hospitalist staff at 12- to 18-month intervals to learn more about their work experience. The team addressed the emotional experience of work, translating empathy to action, professional development, and redesign of structures and processes. Although mutually defining these group core values, 1 specific intervention to alleviate strain was focused on the process of flexible scheduling. Defining these shared values supported implementing a QI tool that created a more predictable and perceived fair schedule resulting in a decline of annual turnover.[35] Another study by Shanafelt and Noseworthy[36] focused on quality of care, patient safety, and patient satisfaction in relation to burnout and linked to prescribing habits, test ordering, the risk of malpractice, and even patient adherence. They concluded that there is a strong case for developing processes whereby organizations invest in provider engagement efforts to reduce burnout and not to assume that burnout was strictly the responsibility of the individual.

A final process measure identified in the literature focuses attention on processes for workplace safety. The media often highlight the friction between physicians and nurses, yet relatively little consideration is given to "nurse-on-nurse lateral violence" in the workplace. It is estimated that anywhere between 45% and 100% of nurses experience incivility and bullying from a nursing colleague.[37] Coworker incivility as a process measure was investigated by Smith and colleagues[38] in a cross-sectional study that used a convenience sample of nearly 300 nurses from 5 hospitals in the southwest United States. The study participants completed an online survey that evaluated the relationship between their work environment and coworker incivility. The nurse work environment was described as "the organizational characteristics of a work setting that facilitate or constrain professional nursing practice." The researchers defined workplace incivility as "the occurrence of low intensity behavior exhibiting an ambiguous intent to harm." Three hospitals in the study were American Nurses Credentialing Center (ANCC) Magnet designated facilities, and 2 sites were in the ANCC Pathway to Excellence Program. The Magnet program distinguishes health care organizations for quality patient care and nursing excellence.[39] The researchers found that a better perception of the nurse work environment was associated with less perceived coworker incivility.[38] Nurse manager attributes were also found to be an influence on work environment associated with incivility, with a positive view of nurse manager leadership ability, and support of nurses associated with lower perceived incivility. The researchers use of Donabedian's model to frame the study proposes that nurse work environment, as an organizational structure, may be associated with the process of coworker incivility. The outcomes of such structure and processes as they relate specifically to nurse burnout and satisfaction require further study.

Outcomes

The last domain of Donabedian's model, identification and assessment of outcomes, clinical quality and safety measures, and satisfaction is critical to measure the association between burnout and quality and safety concerns. Burnout in nursing has been associated with an increased number of adverse events, errors, and patient safety decline.[34,40–42] In the review by Jun and colleagues,[42] they found that emotional exhaustion related to nurse burnout may be associated with adverse patient and organizational outcomes, including increased infection rates related to lower adherence rates of infection control.

Zarei and colleagues[43] evaluated safety climate using questionnaires to measure fatigue, training of nurses, communication with physicians, relationships among nurses, attitude of supervisors, and reporting of errors. The findings show a significant association between safety climate and unit type, job satisfaction, job interest, and stress. The study results also support that improving the safety climate decreases burnout.

Hall and colleagues[41] reported from a systematic review that well-being, as characterized by depression, anxiety, quality of life, stress, and level of burnout, was found to be significantly associated with more self-reported medical errors and near misses.

Several other studies found significant associations between well-being and error (88.9%) as well as an association between burnout and error (83.3%) with high levels of burnout associated with reduced quality of care increased medication errors, increased patient falls, and increased infections.[26,44–46] Cimiotti and colleagues[47] studied infections, burnout, and nurse staffing. Their results found that burnout mediated the relationship between infection and staffing, suggesting that if a nurse reported burnout, every patient added to his or her workload would increase the risk for development of infection. Schlak and colleagues[48] in a cross-sectional study evaluated nurse work environment, burnout, patient outcomes, patient claims data, and Magnet status. They found that processes associated with a positive work environment and Magnet status attenuated the relationship between nurse burnout and certain patient outcomes, such as prolonged patient length of stay, patient mortality, and failure to rescue, concluding that fostering a positive nurse work environment remains a solution for hospitals looking to concurrently improve nurse burnout and quality patient outcomes.

Montgomery and colleagues[49] conducted a cross-sectional electronic survey of acute care nurses using the Copenhagen Burnout Inventory. All burnout dimensions (personal, work-related, and client-related burnout) were significantly correlated with work environment ($r = -0.24$ to -0.57) and were a statistically significant predictor of self-reported medication administration errors (MAEs) ($P<.05$), making them conclude that nurse burnout is a significant factor in predicting MAEs.

A study of Greek RN monitored hand hygiene compliance and measured burnout using the MBI. Analysis of the results showed that controlling for years in practice, burnout was negatively associated with hand hygiene compliance, and nurses reporting higher levels of burnout were less likely to comply with hand hygiene. Given the crucial need to prevent in-hospital infections, this study highlights the need for interventions targeting the prevention of burnout among nursing staff.[50]

THE NATIONAL IMPERATIVE TO REDUCE BURNOUT AND FOCUS ON QUALITY OF CARE

The Agency for Research and Quality (AHRQ) found that provider burnout may impair the providers' ability to maintain safe practices and detect emerging safety threats. AHRQ published findings from a 2019 survey that revealed burnout as a leading patient safety and quality concern among health care organizations. However, only 5% of respondents said that their organization was highly effective at helping staff address burnout.[51] This research enhanced the case for addressing burnout aggressively. However, they recognized that the understanding of the impact of burnout and the effectiveness of interventions to address it are underdeveloped, yet 1 pathway to improved well-being is to ensure that clinicians have the time and resources for their work, fostering workplace engagement.

The Institute for Healthcare Improvement (IHI) developed a *National Action Plan* designed to provide direction to health care leaders, organizations, and associations toward safer care, reduced harm, and recognition that crisis events like the current pandemic call for different approaches to reduce burnout and focus on quality of care. The *Action Plan* calls for increasing open communication and active listening, proactively reaching out to health care workers to see how they are, recognition that help-seeking behaviors are normal, meeting needs of the workforce, and directly asking the workforce what is going well and what is going not so well. IHI also developed a *Guide to Promoting Health Care Workforce Well-Being During and After the COVID-19 Pandemic*.[52] Obviously, the COVID-19 pandemic has exacerbated the already critical issue of health care professional burnout. This guide provides ideas and lessons learned to improve the well-being of the health care workforce, including actions that individuals, leaders, and organizations can take to support the health care workforce during the COVID-19 pandemic and beyond.

In 2020, The Joint Commission (TJC) reported the top 3 issues for health care organizations are mental health and suicide, the aging population, and staff shortages and burnout, citing that clinician burnout has reached alarming proportions according to the research that reports up to half of practicing doctors and nurses experience some manifestations of burnout, and learners in these professions are almost equally affected. TJC developed a New Advisory, *Quick Safety*, Issue 50: "Developing resilience to combat nurse burnout," encouraging health care organizations to address resilience, the process of personal protection from burnout, to protect nurses and other frontline staff.[53] The advisory emphasizes the important role of leadership in creating a positive work environment to empower and motivate nurses and other frontline staff to achieve the best outcomes for patients, staff, and the organization. In addition to supportive actions by leadership, health care organizations can use the following safety actions to help nurses develop resilience in order to combat burnout:

- Provide education for nurses, preceptors, and nurse leaders to identify behaviors caused by burnout and compassion fatigue.
- Improve clinician well-being by measuring it, developing and implementing interventions, and then remeasuring it.
- Offer nurses opportunities to reflect on and learn from practice and other practitioners (eg, positive role models).
- Develop or use current tools for staff to use to anticipate opportunities and problems.
- Work with an internal team to assess if current electronic health record (EHR) system may be customized to optimally support nursing workflow.
- Conduct regular staff meetings with discussions on new organizational policies, processes, and outcomes from higher leadership meetings. Engage nursing input in these meetings.[53]

ORGANIZATIONAL STRATEGIES TO TARGET BURNOUT THAT AFFECT QUALITY AND SAFETY

Patient safety and quality of care are priorities for all health care organizations, so it follows that implementation of strategies that impact patient safety and quality care outcomes are also organizational priorities. The relationship between provider burnout and patient safety and quality of care has been explored and established. As previously discussed, specifically nurse burnout is associated with several organizational factors. These include nurse work environment and staffing[54,55]; lack of clear communication and concern from organizational leadership[56]; perceived lack of organizational support for nurses and other process measures, such as workload, nurse-physician relations, and frontline nursing management[34]; nurse-reported job outcomes and quality of care; and decreased near-miss event reporting and increased adverse event reporting.[4,42,57] Health care organizational efforts that reduce burnout and address the impact of organizational factors associated with nurse burnout have been studied, but more extensive and rigorous research is needed. During the recent COVID-19 pandemic, there has been an increase in the number and innovation in strategies that could be used to proactively identify and reduce burnout, and these are gaining attention.

Identifying Nurse Burnout

Because there is a relationship between nurse burnout and patient safety and quality, acknowledgment and assessment of it is a critical first step for organizations to develop strategies to mitigate it. The tool most widely used to assess burnout is the MBI and includes 3 subscales: emotional exhaustion, depersonalization, and personal accomplishment.[1] The 22-item inventory could be used in abbreviated formats to decrease the length of time to complete and to focus on specific subscales. Periodic assessment of nursing staff communicates an acknowledgment of the phenomenon and the concern the organization has regarding it for not only the well-being of the nursing staff but also the effect burnout has on the culture of safety and patient outcomes.

Leadership Awareness of Burnout and Implications

Once the scope of nurse burnout in the organization is determined, the organization's leadership should demonstrate its commitment to nursing staff well-being and its relationship to patient safety and quality. Leader and manager education and training prepare leaders to recognize that nurse engagement is critical to creating a professional practice environment and preventing burnout.[58] Numerous studies have found a significant association between nurse work environments and staffing on nurse burnout and quality of nursing care.[41] With this knowledge, organizations and organizational leaders may be more compelled to implement changes in the work environment to decrease burnout and increase nurse satisfaction. Initiation of opportunities for increased communication between staff and leaders, such as rounding that includes both staff and managers, was found to be effective in decreasing nurse burnout.[40] Involving staff in organizational decision making, and issues of concern to them on the unit have been shown to improve nurse satisfaction, decrease nurse burnout, and improve patient outcomes.[26,58] Professional nursing practice development in the work environment that allows for nurses' participation in hospital decisions, models of nursing care, relationships between nurses and physicians, and leadership support has been shown to impact quality of care positively.[59] Hughes and colleagues determined that Magnet recognition improved work environment over time, and those hospitals demonstrated better patient safety grades, safety culture scores, and adverse event reporting.[58]

Code Lavender and Lavender Lounges

Providing care to the very sick is stressful, and the COVID-19 pandemic has further highlighted the impact this consistent stress has on health care organizations and those that work in them. Addressing the internal stressors for all staff in health care organizations has required leaders to explore creative strategies to support their work force. Code Lavender and Lavender Lounges have emerged as a strategy to provide a stress-defusing environment for staff. A Code Lavender is a crisis intervention tool that provides a coordinated response from a multidisciplinary team to provide administrative, emotional, and spiritual support to an individual or a team.[60] Some organizations have also created lavender rooms or lavender lounges, which provide a space for staff to take time during their shift to go to the space. The room provides tools for relaxation, such as aromatherapy, guided meditation, and music. They are most importantly a quiet place to reflect and relax uninterrupted. Research on the effectiveness of these interventions is needed.

Schwartz Rounds (Compassion Rounds)

Another innovation that has been proposed by organizations to respond to the high stress of health care delivery is Schwartz rounds, or compassion rounds. These rounds provide a strategy to educate participants on a "shared purpose, interdisciplinary communication, teamwork, and support."[61] Schwartz rounds are usually held for 1 hour monthly and start with a short presentation from someone who reflects on their experience and its impact on them and team members.[62] Others are invited to verbalize the psychosocial and emotional experiences of caring with those who have had similar experiences. In 2018, an evaluation study of these rounds and 11 other strategies to promote health care worker well-being was conducted in the United Kingdom and found that participants that participated in the rounds had a 50% reduction in psychological distress compared with nonparticipants. The participants said they felt less isolation and stress and experienced improvements in well-being, and improvement in relationships with patients and colleagues was seen.[63] More research is needed to determine whether there is a direct cause-and-effect from these new interventions.

"Something Awesome"

Professional interactions, positive communication, and teamwork are associated with improved patient safety, stronger professional engagement, and job satisfaction. Offering opportunities for health care workers to reflect on their day can be a positive first step. One group of hospitalists wanted to improve the emotional experience of their work and instituted an agenda item to their monthly group meetings called "something awesome." This featured a hospitalist sharing a brief story about an "awesome" moment they had while caring for a patient. This strategy, as part of package of more than a dozen interventions implemented by the University of Colorado Hospital Medicine Group to improve well-being over a 5-year period, cut the turnover rate in half and reduced the percentage of those reporting burnout. In addition, the group also reported that the average yearly cost of delivering the interventions was $86,000, but the cost of burnout plus turnover in 2013 was $464,385.[64]

Leadership Development

Work in patient safety has borrowed heavily from similar work in other industries, although some have argued that there are more untapped lessons. Considering that many of the efforts to address and prevent occupational burnout have been performed in other fields, it may also make sense to borrow interventions to address clinician burnout. One such intervention is executive coaching. Gazelle and colleagues[65] used a combination of theory-based principles, drawn from mindfulness, positive psychology, and self-determination theory to develop a leadership coaching program. The program consists of clarification of values, professional and personal goals, along with strategies for accessing individual strengths and reframing negative thinking. These programs are generally delivered in hourly sessions every 1 to 2 weeks for a period of 6 to 12 months. Although data on the effects of leadership coaching in health care settings are limited, coaching has been reported to improve well-being and provide a sound return on investment in other industries.

In the *Journal of the American Medical Association*, Shanafelt and colleagues[66,67] proposed 5 organizational communication strategies for leaders to combat burnout, particularly during the COVID-19 pandemic. They suggest communication strategies should include attention to the following:

- *Hear Me*—Listen and act on lived experience to understand and address concerns to the extent organizations and leaders are able.
- *Protect Me*—Reduce the risk of acquiring COVID-19 and/or being a transmitter to family.

- *Prepare Me*—Provide training and support for high-quality care in different settings.
- *Support Me*—Acknowledge demands and human limitations in times of great patient need.
- *Care for Me*—Provide holistic support for team members and their families, if isolation is required (or other sources of distress occur).

In addition, the American Medical Association has proposed *Five Steps to Promote Joy in Practice* with a foundation in physician leadership development:[64]

1. Understand Burnout at Your Hospital—The common causes of burnout include heavy workload and hours at work, administrative and EHR documentation, lack of autonomy, and a disconnect with leadership.
2. Minimize Burnout and Maximize Engagement—Burnout and engagement are linked to 3 key concepts within the practice of hospital medicine: autonomy, mastery, and purpose.
3. Promote Self-Care and Resilience—Well-being is important; avoid skipping meals, stay hydrated, have healthy snacks available at work, exercise, get enough sleep, and connect with friends and family outside of work.
4. Communicate Frequently with Each Other and Across Specialties—Communication is a foundation of teamwork, and high levels of teamwork have been associated not only with improved patient safety but also with stronger professional engagement and job satisfaction.
5. Recognize and Reward—Develop and implement a culture of reward and recognition to promote collegiality and teamwork.[64]

Employment of a Chief Wellness Officer

Employment of a Chief Wellness Officer (CWO) is the latest strategy being used by organizations to show a commitment to health and wellness. The CWO collects information about the organizational environment, culture, and general feelings of well-being. The role of the CWO is to talk and listen to employees to collect information that can be used to develop, plan, and implement organizational strategies to address burnout. The CWO focuses on raising awareness of employee well-being, including physical, emotional, and behavioral manifestations of burnout. Research on the effectiveness and return on investment of this role needs to be conducted.[68]

Provider Self-Care

Although the previous strategies have all focused on the what the organization can offer, this last category is a collaborative strategy between the work setting and the employee. Health care workers need to collectively address burnout as a professional imperative to improve provider well-being. Be more deliberate in evaluating and cultivating your and your coworkers' emotional health. Individual coworkers who are experiencing burnout may not realize it. All should be alert to signs of burnout among coworkers and colleagues and should talk with each other about how they are feeling at work and balancing work-life with personal life. Identify and speak up if you observe symptoms of stress or burnout in a coworker. If you feel stressed, overwhelmed, or burned out at work, talk with your colleagues about it, seek assistance, and identify a support system. It is important to connect socially and be able to discuss and support each other.

Attend to your own physical health. Ensure that you are getting adequate nutrition, both food and water, during the workday, get adequate sleep, and monitor your activity level. Identify time for yourself to relax and take that time for relaxation. Identify something you like to do and identify time each day to concentrate on that activity and do it! Some examples are reading, writing in a journal, or meditation. Preserve the time. Finally, set aside time throughout the week for physical activity, such as walking, bike riding, or going to the gym or your basement for exercise or yoga. It is well recognized that physical activity can decrease stress levels.

FUTURE DIRECTION

Most of the research on the relationship between burnout and patient safety and quality outcomes has used self-reported perceptions of patient safety, an important but relatively weak outcome measure. As early as 2014, a study of burnout in ICUs in Switzerland concluded the following:

> *[T]he linkage between burnout and safety is driven by both a lack of motivation or energy and impaired cognitive function. In the latter case, they postulate that emotionally exhausted clinicians curtail performance to focus on only the most necessary and pressing tasks. Clinicians with burnout may also have impaired attention, memory, and executive function that decrease their recall and attention to detail. Diminished vigilance, cognitive function, and increased safety lapses place clinicians and patients at higher risk for errors. As burned out clinicians become cynically detached from their work, they may develop negative attitudes toward patients that promote a lack of investment in the clinician–provider interaction, poor communication, and loss of pertinent information for decision-making. Together these factors result in the burned out clinician having impaired capacity to deal with the dynamic and technically complex nature of ICU care effectively.[69]*

The study enrolled 1425 nurses and physicians on 54 ICU teams from 48 different hospitals and evaluated the effect of individual and unit-level burnout scores and clinician ratings of overall safety on standardized mortality ratios and length of stay. Most importantly, the study controlled for unit workload and workload predictability. The higher individual burnout scores were related to poorer overall safety grades. When measured at the unit level, emotional exhaustion (a component of the overall burnout score) was an independent predictor of standardized mortality ratio. These findings support previous studies showing a relationship between burnout and poorer perceptions of safety and represent the strongest evidence to date demonstrating a link between clinician burnout and patient safety outcomes. However, the nature of the relationship remains uncertain, as this type of study cannot determine whether burnout causes higher mortality or whether working in a setting with higher mortality causes burnout. The follow-up question is whether curtailing burnout will improve quality or whether improving quality of care will reduce provider burnout?

SUMMARY

In considering the health care environment, the lens of Donabedian's framework offers a model to evaluate the relationship between patient outcomes, influenced by clinical care delivery structures and processes.[11] Applying Donabedian's model that proposes that adequate and appropriate structures and processes within organizations are necessary to realize optimal outcomes, it is imperative that leadership focuses on those structures and processes to reduce risk of burnout. To mitigate the factors contributing to health care worker burnout, organizations must provide clear communication and sustained implementation of evidence-based processes by which nursing, medical, and allied health professionals can structure their care. Although research continues to evolve, structure and process measures provide a framework to study barriers and facilitators to positive patient and staff outcomes in both crisis and noncrisis circumstances.

It is incumbent upon health care organizations to provide a practice setting where health care professionals feel supported by colleagues, leadership, and collaborators. Inclusion of structural educational programs, including stress management workshops that address psychosocial needs, should be prioritized. Strategies that ensure a thoughtful, organized institutional approach to creating a wellness culture affect and advance well-being at all levels of the organization. The process of transparent, ongoing reciprocal communication between leadership and staff is a key imperative to satisfied nursing workforce. Working collaborations between health care colleagues, for example, physicians and nurses and other professionals, affect the perception of patient-centered care. Organizational attention to enhancing these relationships is essential, as burnout may contribute to the provision of optimal care and outcomes. Health care worker wellness and the effect on patient safety and quality of care are organizational priorities that have become more apparent during the COVID-19 pandemic. Efforts to reduce health care worker burnout will benefit providers, patients, and families, as well as the financial success of the organization.

Berwick, a recognized expert in quality and safety of health care, and Fox[70] commented on Donabedian's model of quality and reported Donabedian saying that "*systems…are enabling mechanisms only. It is the ethical dimension of individuals that is essential to a system's success.*" Donabedian recognized, and worried about, the ascendancy of what he called an "industrial model" of quality improvement. In an interview just before his death, he famously avowed, "*The secret of quality is love. You have to love your patient, you have to love your profession, you have to love your God.*" This reflection sums up the duty that we, as health care professionals, have to focus on reducing burnout in the workplace to ensure quality and safe delivery of health care.

CLINICS CARE POINTS

- Burnout in the workplace can affect the quality and safety of care provided, so every nurse has a professional responsibility to identify symptoms of burnout in themselves and their colleagues.

- Nursing leadership should collaborate with staff to be proactive in assessing burnout in the work setting.

- All staff should identify opportunities to implement innovative strategies to prevent or reduce burnout in the workplace.

DISCLOSURE

The authors have nothing to disclose.

REFERENCES

1. Maslach C, Jackson SE. The measurement of experienced burnout. J organizational Behav 1981;2(2):99–113.
2. World Health Organization (WHO. Burn-out an "occupational phenomenon": International Classification of Diseases. Available at: https://www.who.int/news/item/28-05-2019-burn-out-an-occupational-phenomenon-international-classification-of-diseases. Accessed June 26, 2021.

3. Medscape National Physician Burnout & Suicide Report 2020; the generational divide. Available at: https://www.medscape.com/slideshow/2020-lifestyle-burnout-6012460. Accessed June 29, 2021.

4. Dyrbye LN, Shanafelt TD, Sinsky CA, et al. Burnout among health care professionals: a call to explore and address this underrecognized threat to safe, high-quality care. Washington DC: National Academy of medicine; 2017.

5. BusinessWire. Healthcare worker survey shows they are burned out, sleep deprived, & may quit. 2020. Available at: https://www.businesswire.com/news/home/20201208005303/en/. Accessed on June 29, 2021.

6. Salyers MP, Bonfils KA, Luther L, et al. The relationship between professional burnout and quality and safety in healthcare: a meta-analysis. J Gen Intern Med 2017;32(4):475–82.

7. Carayon P, Gurses AP. Nursing workload and patient safety—a human factors engineering perspective. Chapter 30. In: Hughes RG, editor. Patient safety and quality: an evidence-based handbook for nurses. Rockville (MD): Agency for Healthcare Research and Quality (US); 2008. Available at: https://www.ncbi.nlm.nih.gov/books/NBK2657/.

8. Dall'Ora C, Ball J, Reinius M, et al. Burnout in nursing: a theoretical review. Hum Resour Health 2020;18:41. https://doi.org/10.1186/s12960-020-00469-9.

9. Upadhyay S, Opoku-Agyeman W. Improving healthcare quality in the United States healthcare system: a scientific management approach. J Hosp Adm 2020;9(5):19.

10. Donabedian A. The quality of care. How can it be assessed? JAMA 1988;260(12): 1743–8.

11. Binder C, Torres RE, Elwell D. Use of the Donabedian model as a framework for COVID-19 response at a hospital in suburban Westchester County, New York: a facility-level case report. J Emerg Nurs 2021;47(2):239–55.

12. Tawfik DS, Profit J, Morgenthaler TI, et al. Physician burnout, well-being, and work unit safety grades in relationship to reported medical errors. Mayo Clin Proc 2018;93(11):1571–80.

13. Tawfik DS, Scheid A, Profit J, et al. Evidence relating health care provider burnout and quality of care: a systematic review and meta-analysis. Ann Intern Med 2019; 171(8):555–67.

14. Dyrbye LN, Shanafelt TD, Johnson PO, et al. A cross-sectional study exploring the relationship between burnout, absenteeism, and job performance among American nurses. BMC Nurs 2019;18:57.

15. Dall'ora C, Saville C. Burnout in nursing: what have we learnt and what do we still need to know? Nurs Times 2021;117(2):43–4.

16. Gueritault-Chalvin V, Kalichman SC, Demi A, et al. Work-related stress and occupational burnout in AIDS caregivers: test of a coping model with nurses providing AIDS care. AIDS Care 2000;12(2):149–61.

17. Jameson BE, Bowen F. Use of the worklife and levels of burnout surveys to assess the school nurse work environment. J Sch Nurs 2020;36(4):272–82.

18. Liu Y, Aungsuroch Y. Work stress, perceived social support, self-efficacy, and burnout among Chinese registered nurses. J Nurs Manag 2018;(2):27. https://doi.org/10.1111/jonm.12828.

19. Lowe MA, Prapanjaroensin A, Bakitas MA, et al. An exploratory study of the influence of perceived organizational support, coworker social support, the nursing practice environment, and nurse demographics on burnout in palliative care nurses. J Hosp Palliat Nurs 2020;22(6):465–72.

20. Spence Laschinger HK, Leiter MP. The impact of nursing work environments on patient safety outcomes: the mediating role of burnout/engagement. J Nurs Adm 2006;36(5):259–67.
21. Liu Y, Aungsuroch Y. Factors influencing nurse-assessed quality nursing care: a cross-sectional study in hospitals. J Adv Nurs 2018;74(4):935–45.
22. Garcia CL, Abreu LC, Ramos JLS, et al. Influence of burnout on patient safety: systematic review and meta-analysis. Medicina (Kaunas) 2019;55(9):553.
23. West CP, Dyrbye LN, Shanafelt TD. Physician burnout: contributors, consequences and solutions. J Intern Med 2018;283(6):516–29.
24. Alves DF, Silva D, Guirardello EB. Nursing practice environment, job outcomes and safety climate: a structural equation modeling analysis. J Nurs Management 2016;25(1):46–55.
25. Profit J, Sharek PJ, Amspoker AB, et al. Burnout in the NICU setting and its relation to safety culture. BMJ Qual Saf 2014;23(10):806–13.
26. Van Bogaert P, Timmermans O, Weeks SM, et al. Nursing unit teams matter: impact of unit-level nurse practice environment, nurse work characteristics, and burnout on nurse reported job outcomes, and quality of care, and patient adverse events–a cross-sectional survey. Int J Nurs Stud 2014;51(8):1123–34.
27. Guirardello EB. Impact of critical care environment on burnout, perceived quality of care and safety attitude of the nursing team. Rev Lat Am Enfermagem 2017;25: e2884.
28. Shanafelt TD, Gorringe G, Menaker R, et al. Impact of organizational leadership on physician burnout and satisfaction. Mayo Clin Proc 2015;90(4):432–40.
29. Linzer M, Poplau S, Grossman E, et al. A cluster randomized trial of interventions to improve work conditions and clinician burnout in primary care: results from the Healthy Work Place (HWP) Study. J Gen Intern Med 2015;30(8):1105–11.
30. Sikka R, Morath JM, Leape L. The quadruple aim: care, health, cost and meaning in work. BMJ Qual Saf 2015;24(10):608–10.
31. Rathert C, Williams ES, Linhart H. Evidence for the quadruple aim: a systematic review of the literature on physician burnout and patient outcomes. Med Care 2018;56(12):976–84.
32. Bodenheimer T, Sinsky C. From triple to quadruple aim: care of the patient requires care of the provider. Ann Fam Med 2014;12(6):573–6.
33. Park JY, Hwang JI. J Korean Acad Nurs 2021;51(1):27–39.
34. Liu X, Zheng J, Liu K, et al. Hospital nursing organizational factors, nursing care left undone, and nurse burnout as predictors of patient safety: a structural equation modeling analysis. Int J Nurs Stud 2018;86:82–9.
35. Zarefsky M. Success story: physicians and leaders work together to achieve top performance and joy in patient care. AMA Steps Forward 2020. Available at: https://edhub.ama-assn.org/steps-forward/module/2776939. Accessed on June 29, 2021.
36. Shanafelt TD, Noseworthy JH. Executive leadership and physician well-being: nine organizational strategies to promote engagement and reduce burnout. Mayo Clin Proc 2017;92(1):129–46.
37. Edmonson C, Zelonka C. Our own worst enemies: the nurse bullying epidemic. Nurs Adm Q 2019;43(3):274–9.
38. Smith JG, Morin KH, Lake ET. Association of the nurse work environment with nurse incivility in hospitals. J Nurs Manag 2018;26(2):219–26.
39. American Nurses Credentialing Center. About ANCC. 2017 [WWW document]. Available at: http://www.nursecredentialing.org/About-ANCC. Accessed May 18, 2021.

40. Alves DF, Guirardello EB. Safety climate, emotional exhaustion and job satisfaction among Brazilian paediatric professional nurses. Int Nurs Rev 2016;63(3): 328–35.
41. Hall LH, Johnson J, Watt I, et al. Healthcare staff wellbeing, burnout, and patient safety: a systematic review. PLoS One 2016;11(7):e0159015.
42. Jun J, Ojemeni MM, Kalamani R, et al. Relationship between nurse burnout, patient and organizational outcomes: systematic review. Int J Nurs Stud 2021;119: 103933.
43. Zarei E, Khakzad N, Reniers G, et al. On the relationship between safety climate and occupational burnout in healthcare organizations. Saf Sci 2016;89:1–10. https://doi.org/10.1016/j.ssci.2016.05.011.
44. Poghosyan L, Clarke SP, Finlayson M, et al. Nurse burnout and quality of care: cross-national investigation in six countries. Res Nurs Health 2010;33(4):288–98.
45. Van Bogaert P, Clarke S, Roelant E, et al. Impacts of unit-level nurse practice environment and burnout on nurse-reported outcomes: a multilevel modelling approach. J Clin Nurs 2010;19(11–12):1664–74.
46. Van Bogaert P, Kowalski C, Weeks SM, et al. The relationship between nurse practice environment, nurse work characteristics, burnout and job outcome and quality of nursing care: a cross-sectional survey. Int J Nurs Stud 2013; 50(12):1667–77.
47. Cimiotti JP, Aiken LH, Sloane DM, et al. Nurse staffing, burnout, and health care-associated infection. Am J Infect Control 2012;40(6):486–90 [published correction appears in Am J Infect Control. 2012 Sep;40(7):680].
48. Schlak AE, Aiken LH, Chittams J, et al. Leveraging the work environment to minimize the negative impact of nurse burnout on patient outcomes. Int J Environ Res Public Health 2021;18:610. https://doi.org/10.3390/ijerph18020610.
49. Montgomery AP, Azuero A, Baernholdt M, et al. Nurse burnout predicts self-reported medication administration errors in acute care hospitals. J Healthc Qual 2021;43(1):13–23.
50. Manomenidis G, Panagopoulou E. Montgomery. Job burnout reduces hand hygiene compliance among nursing staff. J Patient Saf 2019;15(1):e70–3.
51. AHRQ 2019 Annual Patient Safety & Quality Industry Outlook. Kennesaw (GA): Patient safety & quality healthcare (PSQH), psqh.com/intelligence.
52. Institute for Healthcare Improvement. A guide to promoting health care workforce well-being during and after the COVID-19 pandemic. Boston, Massachusetts: Institute for Healthcare Improvement; 2020. Available at: https://wellbeingtrust.org/wp-content/uploads/2020/12/IHI-Guide-to-Promoting-Health-Care-Workforce-Well-Being.pdf. Accessed on July 2, 2021.
53. The Joint Commission. Quick safety: developing resilience to combat nurse burnout. July 15, 2019. Issue 50.
54. Nantsupawat A, Srisuphan W, Kunaviktikul W, et al. Impact of nurse work environment and staffing on hospital nurse and quality of care in Thailand. J Nurs Scholarsh 2011;43(4):426–32.
55. Kirwan M, Matthews A, Scott A. The impact of the work environment of nurses on patient safety outcomes: a multi-level modelling approach. Int J Nurs Stud 2013; 50(2):253–63. https://doi.org/10.1016/j.ijnurstu.2012.08.020.
56. O'Mahoney N. Nurse burnout and the working environment. Emerg Nurse. 19, 5, 30-37. doi:
57. Nantsupawat A, Nantsupawat R, Kunaviktikul W, et al. Nurse burnout, nurse-reported quality of care, and patient outcomes in Thai hospitals. J Nurs Scholarsh 2016;48(1):83–90.

58. Institute of Medicine (U.S.). Committee on the Work Environment for Nurses and Patient Safety. Ann Page. Keeping patients safe: transforming the work environment of nurses. Washington, DC: National Academies Press; 2004.

59. Olds D, Aiken L, Cimiotti J, et al. Association of nurse work environment and safety climate on patient mortality: a cross-sectional study. Int J Nurs Stud 2017;74:155–1621.

60. Stone S. Code Lavender: a tool for staff support. Nursing 2018;15.

61. Lown BA, Manning CF. The Schwartz center rounds: evaluation of an interdisciplinary approach to enhancing patient-centered communication, teamwork, and provider support. Acad Med 2010;85(6):1073–81.

62. Robert G, Philippou J, Leamy M. Exploring the adoption of Schwartz center rounds as an organisational innovation to improve staff well-being in England, 2009–2015. BMJ Open 2017;7. https://doi.org/10.1136/bmjopen-2016-014326.

63. Taylor C, Xyrichis A, Leamy M. Can Schwartz Centre rounds support healthcare staff with emotional challenges at work, and how do they compare with other interventions aimed at providing similar support? BMJ Open 2018;8. https://doi.org/10.1136/bmjopen-2018-024254.

64. Cyrus R, Fitterman N, Barrett E, Van Opstal E, Brown M, Jin J. Hospitalist well being maximize engagement and minimize burnout for hospitalists. AMA Steps Forward. 2019. Available at: https://edhub.ama-assn.org/%20on%2006/27/2021.

65. Gazelle G, Liebschutz JM, Riess H. Physician burnout: coaching a way out. J Gen Intern Med 2015;30(4):508–13.

66. Shanafelt T, Ripp J, Trockel M. Understanding and addressing sources of anxiety among health care professionals during the COVID-19 pandemic. JAMA 2020; 323(21):2133–4.

67. Shanafelt T, Trockel M, Ripp J, et al. Building a program on well-being: key design considerations to meet the unique needs of each organization. Acad Med 2019; 94(2):156–61.

68. Lazarus A. Chief Wellness Officer: new opportunity, necessary role 2019. Available at: https://www.healthaffairs.org/do/10.1377/hblog20181025.308059/full/. Accessed May 30, 2021.

69. Welp A, Meier LL, Manser T. Emotional exhaustion and workload predict clinician-rated and objective patient safety. Front Psychol 2015;5:1573. https://doi.org/10.3389/fpsyg.2014.01573.

70. Berwick D, Fox DM. Evaluating the quality of medical care": Donabedian's classic article 50 years later. Milbank Q 2016;94(2):237–41.

The Influence of Leadership Style and Nurse Empowerment on Burnout

Vincent P. Hall, PhD, RN, CNE[a],*,
Kathleen M. White, PhD, RN, NEA-BC, FAAN[b],
Jeanne Morrison, PhD, MSN[c]

KEYWORDS

• Leadership style • Nurse empowerment • Burnout

KEY POINTS

• Burnout is a syndrome that significantly affects the nursing workforce.
• Burnout affects the physical, psychological, and emotional health of nurses and can have considerable negative implications for nurse retention, patient safety, patient outcomes, and health care organizations.
• Nurse leaders and their leadership style can play a significant role in facilitating a healthy work environment, increasing a sense of empowerment among nursing staff, and decreasing burnout.

OVERVIEW OF BURNOUT

Burnout is a syndrome that is characterized by 3 distinct but interrelated dimensions, emotional exhaustion, cynicism or depersonalization, and a perceived lack of personal accomplishment. Typically, emotional exhaustion is seen as the first sign of burnout and refers to the intense feelings of lack of physical and emotional resources to draw on as a result of chronic and/or sustained feelings of being overwhelmed or exposed to suffering and stress on the job. The emotionally exhausted clinician is overwhelmed by work to the point of feeling fatigued, unable to face the demands of the job, and unable to engage with others. Following this emotional exhaustion and continued exposure to job stressors, the individual develops a sense of detachment and cynicism or depersonalization from his/her work or aspects of the job. The development of the sense of cynical detachment from work view people, especially patients, as objects. Finally, as a result of emotional exhaustion and feelings of depersonalization, the individual begins to experience feelings of incompetence or lack of personal achievement at work, the third dimension of burnout.[1] Fatigue,

[a] Walden University, 56 Ravencroft Lane, Asheville, NC 28803, USA; [b] Johns Hopkins University, 2850 Pebble Beach Drive, Ellicott City, MD 21042, USA; [c] Walden University, 23 Elks Lake Road, Hattiesburg, MS 39401, USA
* Corresponding author.
E-mail address: vincent.hall@mail.waldenu.edu

Nurs Clin N Am 57 (2022) 131–141
https://doi.org/10.1016/j.cnur.2021.11.009
0029-6465/22/© 2021 Elsevier Inc. All rights reserved.
nursing.theclinics.com

exhaustion, and detachment coalesce such that clinicians no longer feel effective at work because they have lost a sense of their ability to contribute meaningfully. According to Maslach, Jackson, and Leiter, burnout has 6 main causes: (1) an unsustainable workload; (2) employees' perceived lack of control in the work setting; (3) insufficient rewards for effort; (4) lack of a supportive work community; (5) perceived lack of fairness in the organization; and (6) mismatched set of values and skills.[2]

In the past few years, the growing prevalence of burnout syndrome among health care workers has gained attention as a potential threat to health care quality and patient safety. In late 2015, the Mayo Clinic conducted study in partnership with the American Medical Association and found that more than half of American physicians now have at least one sign of burnout, which was a 9% increase from the same group's prior study conducted 3 years earlier.

In the fall of 2020, the American Association of Physician Leadership in collaboration with several partners and supported by the Harvard Business Review conducted a survey to measure health care employees' perceptions of work-setting qualities that affect their work engagement or the state of burnout during COVID-19. They gathered 1500 responses from 46 countries supporting that burnout is a global problem. The survey found that

- 89% of respondents said their work life was getting worse
- 85% said their well-being had declined
- 56% said their job demands had increased
- 62% of the people who were struggling to manage their workloads had experienced burnout "often" or "extremely often" in the previous 3 months
- 57% of employees felt that the pandemic had a "large effect on" or "completely dominated" their work
- 55% of all respondents did not feel that they had been able to balance their home and work life—with 53% specifically citing homeschooling
- 25% felt unable to maintain a strong connection with family, 39% with colleagues, and 50% with friends
- Only 21% rated their well-being as "good," and a mere 2% rated it as "excellent"[3]

Burnout is and has been a significant problem for the nursing profession for years, and the nursing literature is replete with studies that report burnout is a common problem among nurses. Shah and colleagues conducted a secondary analysis of the 2018 National Sample Survey of Registered Nurses in the United States to determine national estimates of nurse burnout and associated factors that may put nurses at risk for burnout. They found that among nurses who reported leaving their job in 2017, 31.5% reported burnout as a reason, with lower proportions of nurses reporting burnout in the West (16.6%) and higher proportions in the Southeast (30.0%). In addition, survey respondents who reported leaving or considering leaving their job due to burnout reported a stressful work environment (68.6% and 59.5%, respectively) and inadequate staffing (63.0% and 60.9%, respectively).[4] In a 2021 systematic review of the literature, D'All Ora and Saville found significant reports that adverse job characteristics are associated with burnout in nursing, with potential severe consequences of burnout for both staff and patients.[5]

THE CHALLENGE OF BURNOUT FOR NURSE LEADERS

Between one-third and one-half of US clinicians experience burnout, and addressing this syndrome requires systemic changes by health care organizations, educational institutions, and all levels of government, according to a new report from the National Academy of Medicine.[6] Victor J. Dzau, the president of the National Academy of Medicine President, was quoted as saying "system-level solutions aimed at reducing or preventing burnout for clinicians of all types, across all workplaces and career stages, are essential to supporting a high-functioning health system and satisfactory patient experience. Health care leaders at all levels must take urgent action to uphold clinician well-being as a fundamental value that is essential to the fulfilment of their missions."[7] The report, *Taking Action Against Clinician Burnout: A Systems Approach to Professional Well-Being,* outlines goals for health care organizational leaders to be proactive and identify the presence of burnout, take steps to prevent and mitigate provider burnout, and foster feelings of professional well-being and joy in their work. The 2021 American Hospital Association Environmental Scan reported the emotional health and well-being of staff is the top challenge for nurse leaders during the pandemic.[8]

Burnout is associated with a wide range of physical, emotional, and behavioral symptoms frequently reported in the literature that nurse leaders must be alert to and proactively identify in their staff. Common physical symptoms include tiredness, change in appetite, change in sleep patterns, headache, and muscle aches. Prevalent emotional symptoms often include a sense of hopelessness and helplessness feelings of self-doubt and lack of job satisfaction. Concerning behavioral symptoms of burnout include anxiety, depression, lack of motivation, substance use and abuse, insomnia, and dissatisfaction, leading to conflicts.

The presence of these signs and symptoms of burnout in the workplace leads to deterioration in the quality and safety of the health care work environment associated with negative clinical outcomes such as low patient satisfaction, poor communication with patients and staff, poor patient engagement, and self-reported increase in medical errors.[9] In addition, reduced work performance, low employee morale, absenteeism, lower organizational commitment, and increase in job turnover are often observed work consequences.[10,11] These ultimately result in perceived lack of autonomy by clinicians, employee disconnection with leadership, and higher costs to the organization.[12]

From June to September 2020, Mental Health America hosted a survey to listen to the experiences of health care workers during COVID-19. The respondents said they were stressed out and stretched too thin: 93% of health care workers were experiencing stress, 86% reported experiencing anxiety, 77% reported frustration, 76% reported exhaustion and burnout, and 75% said they were overwhelmed. Emotional exhaustion was the most commonly reported answer on how the health care workers were feeling over the previous 3 months (82%), followed by trouble with sleep (70%), physical exhaustion (68%), and work-related dread (63%). More than half of the respondents reported that they had changes in appetite (57%), physical symptoms such as headache or stomachache (56%), feelings of compassion fatigue (52%), heightened awareness or attention to being exposed (52%), and were questioning their career path (55%). Fifty-four percent of respondents reported experiencing burnout and almost half (49%) reported a heavy or increased workload as a major stressor in the previous 3 months.[13] Nurse leaders face important and specific challenges in supporting staff and mitigating burnout to address the current moral distress and emotional exhaustion during the Covid-19 pandemic and beyond.[14]

Finally, burnout is viewed as a threat to patient safety. Burnout among health care providers has been associated with poor patient and provider outcomes. Providers with burnout are more likely to report lower patient safety in their organizations and admit to or self-report having made mistakes or delivering less than optimal patient care.[15]

Addressing burnout is a major challenge and critical priority for today's health care organizations, and leadership style has generally been identified as a means to reduce burnout, yet it is unclear whether some leadership styles are more effective than others at mitigating burnout.[16] Leadership style is the manner and characteristics exhibited by an individual to influence others to act and achieve a common goal. There are many different leadership styles, and a better understanding of the leadership styles may provide guidance on opportunities and strategies to reduce employee burnout.

LEADERSHIP STYLES

A nursing leader's work environment is full of opportunities and challenges. The nursing profession's challenges include increased acuity level of patients, high physical demands, enhanced technology, and decreased job satisfaction, resulting in burnout. Because of these challenges, nurses may experience a lack of empowerment, which may lead to burnout.[17,18] As noted earlier, this can have a significant impact on patient outcomes and the goals of an organization.[19]

Empowerment is an effective leadership tool that can help lessen the effect of stress and burnout.[17] Nursing leaders must learn to create an environment that promotes a positive work climate that empowers employees. Effective leadership styles can provide the necessary skills to keep the staff empowered.[20] This section examines 3 leadership styles, transformational leadership, resonant leadership, and authentic leadership, and their relationship to structural and psychological empowerment.

Empowerment

Staff experience empowerment when provided with the opportunities, resources, and authority to do their job.[21] Kanter's early view of the definition of power is the "ability to get things done, to mobilize resources."[6(p166)] Kanter suggests that employees will increase their power when provided with enhanced opportunities for growth, information, support, and resources within an organization.[22,23] Empowerment is a shared power relationship between the leader and employee. A dual perspective has examined empowerment, one being structural empowerment and the other being psychological empowerment.[17,24]

Structural empowerment refers to nurses receiving support from leaders, having the necessary resources and information to complete the job and growth opportunities, which include infrastructures, company policies, knowledge sharing, organizational changes, feedback from peers and supervisors, career advancement, open communication, and time and financial resources. When nurses are given a solid structure within an organization, they feel empowered to complete the organizational goals in a meaningful way.[21,25,26] Structural empowerment is a critical piece for a positive work environment.[20]

Psychological empowerment can act as a motivational tool affecting an individual's behavior.

Spreitzer[27] suggests psychological empowerment has 4 dimensions:

- Meaning: does the employee feel their contribution to the organization has meaning?
- Competence: does the employee complete work activities with proficiency?
- Self-determination: does the employee have a sense of autonomy when starting and completing tasks?
- Impact: is the employee making a difference?

Transformational Leadership

The transformational leadership theory has been a dominant nursing theory for the past several decades. Burns provided the foundation for the transformational theory in 1978, and it was further developed by Bass in 1985, explaining how leaders affect employees. This theory suggests meeting the higher needs of employees who will eventually take on leadership roles.[28,29] The theory sets clear guidelines and expectations, encouraging and motivating employees.[21]

Transformational leaders (TL) provide resources and opportunities for employees to grow in a highly competitive workplace. TL encourages employees to challenge themselves and take the extra steps for personal and organizational goals.[26] Leaders set clear guidelines and expectations while encouraging and motivating employees.[30] The 4 elements of transformational leadership include the following:[26]

- Idealized influence: leaders engaging behavior instill trust and connection with employees.
- Inspirational communication: leaders communicate a clear vision for the organization. Their communication is positive and encouraging, which builds self-confidence in employees.
- Intellectual stimulation: leaders encourage employees to challenge themselves and be creative with a new way of thinking.
- Individual consideration: leaders meet the needs of employees, acting as a mentor and providing individual support.

Boamah and colleagues suggest that transformational leaders positively affect structural and psychological empowerment.[30] When a transformational leader uses empowering behaviors as described in the 4 elements of a transformational leader, this feeling of empowerment will ultimately lead to increased work engagement.[21,26,31] Transformational leaders communicate an organization's vision while inspiring and motivating the employees to achieve this mutual goal. This type of leadership produces employee satisfaction, innovation, and commitment and improves organizational performance. Transformational leaders elevate their employee's self-efficacy by giving them a purpose and direction and at the same time showing confidence in their ability to achieve goals.[21,31,32]

Transformational nurse leaders are generally highly involved with their staff. They treat staff as individuals, listen to concerns, and spend time teaching and coaching their nursing staff to assist them develop their skills and strengths as professionals. Research provides support that a TL style can promote greater job satisfaction among nursing staff rather that other styles such as laissez-faire or passive-avoidant styles.[33] Research also indicates that along with improved job satisfaction, TL as a leadership style may have an environmental protective factor that reduces burnout and turnover as well as the impact of depressive symptoms on feelings of personal accomplishment.[34] TL is significantly associated with promoting a healthy work environment for nurses, which is associated with higher nurse engagement and lower nurse burnout.[35] In addition, TL has been found to promote stronger teamwork among nurses, facilitate nurse well-being and quality of care, and provide a climate that increases the meaningfulness of work.[18,36]

Resonant Leadership

According to Boyatzis and McKee, resonance leadership (RL) style is relationally focused.[37] This type of leadership style is based on the theory of Emotional

Intelligence (EI). EI is a combination of interpersonal and emotional competencies that influence personal behavior and relationships.[38]

These 2 EI competencies are categorized into 2 categories: personal and social. Personal includes self-awareness and self-management. Social includes social awareness and relationship management.[38]

- *Self-awareness* is understanding one's own emotions, strength, motivation, and limitations.
- *Self-management* is making correct decisions based on one's self-awareness.
- *Social awareness* is understanding others and having empathy.
- *Relationship management* combines self-awareness, self-management, and social awareness and applying them to relationship management.

RL's 3 core qualities are based on the competencies of emotional intelligence.[37]

- *Mindfulness* is having an awareness of oneself and being understanding and mindful of others.
- *Hope* is having a vision for the future.
- *Compassion* is caring for oneself and others.

Successful resonant leaders must first have self-awareness and understand their feelings before learning how to motivate and connect with employees. RLs are aware of the feelings and the perceptions of their employees.[37,39] They lead by developing strong and trusting relationships with others. They are empathetic and able to read people in groups effectively and accurately. Resonant leaders develop solid and trusting relationships with others. They make their employees feel valued and essential, using hope, optimism, and encouragement with employees. RL supports innovative ideas from others.[25,37]

Structural empowerment is a principal factor when creating a positive work environment for nurses.[20] Resonant leaders focus on mindfulness and self-care to create an effective work environment for staff.[37,38] The main attributes of a resonant leader with emotional intelligence understand their skills and building relationships within an organization. With structural empowerment, building effective relationships include sharing information, effective communication, positive career advancement, and resources needed. This feeling of structural empowerment will lead to increased job satisfaction.[39]

Resonant leaders with EI give hope, compassion, and empathy to others. RL enhances psychological empowerment and increased meaningfulness in the work environment. The staff feels psychologically empowered with a connection to their organization. They have the sense of leader's support in starting and completing tasks and making a difference in the organization.[39,40]

As a positive relational leadership style, RL has the potential for long-term effectiveness because of the leader's focus on empathy, building trust, self-care, and the ability of the leader to develop and maintain a positive work environment over time.[25] As an emerging leadership style, very few studies have examined resonant leadership in nursing and health care and its impact on burnout. Research has suggested that the RL of nurse managers has a significant direct and an indirect effect on the job satisfaction of nurses through structural empowerment.[39] In addition, there is evidence that an RL style that fosters an empowering work environment can facilitate lower levels of incivility and burnout and increase job satisfaction.[40]

Authentic Leadership

Authentic leadership (AL) shares some of the same concepts as other leadership theories, such as transformational and servant leadership. An authentic leader's primary goal is to guide the employees to develop a sense of self.[24] With authentic leadership, high-level communication exists between the leader and staff. Because of the leader-member exchange with authentic leadership, AL affects the self-regulated behaviors of both leader and employee.[30,40]

Walumbwa suggests AL consists of leadership behavior that promotes a positive ethical climate in the organization.[41] This climate stimulates the psychological empowerment of both the leader and nursing staff. This empowerment creates a shared sense of "us" between the leader and employee. Authentic leadership has 4 primary characteristics:[40–44]

- First, *a person with self-awareness* understands one's emotions, goals, knowledge, and talents, as well as weaknesses.
- *Relational transparency* is communicating with openness and clarity.
- *Internalized moral perspective* is alignment between the value of the leader and ethical conduct.
- *Balanced processing* refers to leaders who examine all situations/evidence before making decisions.

According to Dwyer and colleagues, AL positively correlates with structural empowerment. AL provides the staff nurses with the necessary resources and the support to do their job effectively.[19] ALs are transparent in their communication with the staff. The vision of the organization is presented to employees with openness and clarity. They encourage the sharing of information with other members of the organization. Employees tend to mirror their leader's AL behaviors, which contribute to a higher level of engagement and performance by the staff.[19,42,43]

The characteristics of an authentic leader, such as self-awareness, internalized moral perspective, and balanced processing, align with the psychological empowerment of staff. Authentic leadership encourages the personal growth of nurses. The nurses' opinions and viewpoints are valued regardless of their position in the organization. This collaboration stimulates the collective intelligence of the group. Staff nurses are recognized and praised for their contributions. The leader's ethical values are understood by the staff and help create a trusting relationship.[24,43]

AL is increasingly being recognized as a leadership style that can positively influence the nursing work environment.[45] Further, there is a growing body of research that indicates AL may help reduce burnout among nursing staff and promote empowerment in the workplace. AL has been found to create supportive work environments that may decrease or discourage the incidence of bullying and burnout and thus possibly improving nurse satisfaction and retention.[46,47] AL has been found to have a positive effect on work life (person-job fit) and therefore positively affecting nurses' confidence in their ability to cope with the demands of the job, which can potentially lead to lower rates of burnout.[48] Other research has shown that authentic leaders tend to support or shape working environments where norms of civility guide acceptable behavior in the workplace. The creation of civility norms can help support health working conditions that foster satisfaction, decrease incidence of incivility, and thereby decrease burnout.[45] Finally, there is evidence that AL can have a positive impact on structural empowerment, providing nurses with a supportive environment that fosters job satisfaction, reduces burnout, and improves the quality of patient care.[49]

SUMMARY

In addition to the significant impact on the physical and emotional health of nurses, burnout as a syndrome can lead to reduced work performance, low employee morale, absenteeism, lower organizational commitment, and increases in job turnover that result in higher costs to the organization.[10–12] Negative clinical outcomes such as low patient satisfaction, poor communication with patients and staff, poor patient engagement, and self-reported increase in medical errors can also occur.[9] However, there are additional workforce and demographic changes to consider when examining the impact of burnout on the nursing profession. It is projected that a shortage of registered nurses (RNs) will evolve across the United States (US) between 2016 and 2030. At the same time, it is projected that the number of US residents aged 65 years and older will be 82 million. A larger number of older adults will increase the need for geriatric care along with care for individuals with chronic illness and comorbidities. Although the RN workforce is expected to grow from 3 million in 2019 to 3.3 million in 2029, with the average age of an RN being 50 years, it is also expected that 175,900 openings for RNs will occur each year through 2029 when nurse retirements and workforce exits are factored into the number of nurses needed.[50] Therefore, it becomes essential that health care institutions recruit and retain enough nurses to care for an aging population with increased and complex nursing and health care needs.

It is recognized that a significant challenge to health care quality and the recruitment and retention of nurses in the next 10 years is the increasing prevalence of burnout within the nursing profession.[51,52] Although issues within the nursing practice environment such as poor communication, demanding workloads, and lack of autonomy can lead to burnout, there is increasing evidence that nurse leaders and their leadership style can play a significant role in facilitating a healthy work environment and decreasing burnout.[51]

The leadership styles described in this article come from different theoretic perspectives but each reflect a positive relational leadership style. In addition, they share some common characteristics in that each style values: (1) effective communication that supports the open sharing of information and consideration of different viewpoints, (2) establishing and supporting trusting relationships, and (3) motivating others to develop as individuals and engaging them to work for common goals.[33] All 3 leadership styles, transformational, resonant, and authentic, also promote the empowerment of staff nurses.[17] Nurses who feel empowered are inspired to achieve both personal and professional goals. Nurse leaders are essential in developing and fostering positive work environments that retain an empowered and motivated workforce. Positive and relational leadership styles can improve nurses' job satisfaction, organizational commitment, and intent to stay in their position while concurrently reducing emotional exhaustion and burnout.[33]

CLINICS CARE POINTS

- Nurses in leadership positions should be aware of potential behavioral changes in their nursing staff that may indicate burnout such as reduced work performance, low morale, absenteeism, and signs of fatigue or exhaustion.

- Common physical symptoms of burnout can include tiredness, changes in appetite, changes in sleep patterns, headaches, and muscle aches, whereas emotional symptoms often include a sense of hopelessness and helplessness, feelings of self-doubt, and lack of job satisfaction.

- Nursing care environments that support effective communication, trusting relationships, and a motivational and engaging atmosphere can assist in the reduction of burnout in nursing staff.

DISCLOSURE

The authors have nothing to disclose.

REFERENCES

1. Maslach C, Jackson SE. The measurement of experienced burnout. J Occup Behav 1981;2:99–113.
2. Maslach C, Leiter M, Jackson SE. Making a significant difference with burnout interventions: Researcher and practitioner collaboration. J Organizational Behav 2012;33:296–300.
3. Moss J. Beyond burned out. American Association of Physician Leadership; 2021. Available at: https://www.physicianleaders.org/news/beyond-burned-out. Accessed July 3, 2021.
4. Shah MK, Gandrakota N, Cimiotti JP, et al. Prevalence of and factors associated with nurse burnout in the US. JAMA Netw Open 2021;4(2):e2036469.
5. Dall'Ora C, Saville C. Burnout in nursing: what have we learnt and what is still unknown? Nurs Times 2021;117(2):43–4.
6. National Academies of Sciences, Engineering, and Medicine. Taking action against clinician burnout: a systems Approach to professional well-being. Washington, DC: The National Academies Press; 2019. https://doi.org/10.17226/25521. Available at:.
7. National Academies of Sciences, Engineering and Medicine. To Ensure High-Quality Patient Care, the Health Care System Must Address Clinician Burnout Tied to Work and Learning Environments, Administrative Requirements News Release. October 23, 2019. Available at: https://www.nationalacademies.org/news/2019/10/to-ensure-high-quality-patient-care-the-health-care-system-must-address-clinician-burnout-tied-to-work-and-learning-environments-administrative-requirements. Accessed July 3, 2021.
8. American Hospital Association. 2021 Environmental Scan. Chicago (IL): American Hospital Association; 2020. Available at: https://www.aha.org/environmentalscan. Accessed July 3, 2021.
9. Salyers MP, Flanagan ME, Firmin R, et al. Clinicians' perceptions of how burnout affects their work. Psychiatr Serv 2015;66(2):204–7.
10. Bakker AB, Demerouti E, Sanz-Verget AS. Burnout and Work Engagement: The JD–R Approach. Annu Rev Organizational Psychol Organizational Behav 2014; 1(1):389–411.
11. Salvagioni DAJ, Melanda FN, Mesas AE, et al. Physical, psychological and occupational consequences of job burnout: A systematic review of prospective studies. PLoS One 2017;12(10):e0185781.
12. Cyrus R, Fitterman N, Barrett E, et al. Hospitalist Well-Being: maximize engagement and minimize burnout for hospitalists, 2019, AMA Steps Forward. Available at: Hospitalist Well-Being | Professional Well-being | AMA STEPS Forward | AMA Ed Hub (ama-assn.org). Accessed June 27, 2021.
13. Mental Health America. The mental health of health care workers in COVID-19 2020. Available at: https://mhanational.org/mental-health-healthcare-workers-covid-19. Accessed July 3, 2021.
14. Sriharan A, West KJ, Almost J, et al. COVID-19-related occupational burnout and moral distress among nurses: a rapid scoping review. Nurs Leadersh (Tor Ont) 2021;34(1):7–19. Available at: https://doi-org.dbproxy.lasalle.edu/10.12927/cjnl.2021.26459.
15. Montgomery AP, Azuero A, Baernholdt MB, et al. Nurse burnout predicts self-reported medication administration errors in acute care hospitals. J Healthc Qual 2020;43(1):13–23.

16. Kelly RJ, Hearld LR. Burnout and leadership style in behavioral health care: a literature review. J Behav Health Serv Res 2020;47(4):581–600.

17. Nursalam N, Fibriansari RD, Yuwomo MH, et al. Development of an empowerment model for burnout syndrome and quality of nursing work life in Indonesia. Int J Nurs Sci 2018;5:390–5.

18. Wu X, Hayter M, Lee AJ, et al. Positive spiritual climate supports transformational leadership as means to reduce nursing burnout and intent to leave. J Nurs Manag 2020;28(4):804–13.

19. Dwyer PA, Revell SM, Sethares KA, et al. The influence of psychological capital, authentic leadership in preceptors, and structural empowerment on new graduate nurse burnout and turnover intent. Appl Nurs Res 2019;48:37–44.

20. Larrabee J, Janne M, Ostrow CL, et al. Predicting registered nurse job satisfaction and intent to leave. J Nurs Adm 2003;33(5):271–83.

21. Monje Amor A, Abeal Vázquez JP, Faíña JA. Transformational leadership and work engagement: Exploring the mediating role of structural empowerment. Eur Manag J 2020;38(1):169–78.

22. Kanter RM. Men and women of the corporation. New York: Basic Books; 1977.

23. Kanter RM. Men and women of the corporation. 2nd edition. New York: Basic Books; 1993.

24. Beiranvand M, Beiranvand S, Beiranvand S, et al. Explaining the effect of authentic and ethical leadership on psychological empowerment of nurses. J Nurs Manag 2021;00:1–10.

25. Baker K. Review: The influence of resonant leadership on the structural empowerment and job satisfaction of registered nurses. J Res Nurs 2015;20(7):623–4.

26. Schermuly CC, Meyer B. Transformational leadership psychological empowerment and flow at work. Eur J Work Organ Psychol 2020;29(5):740–52.

27. Spreitzer GM. Psychological empowerment in the workplace: Dimensions, measurement, and validation. Acad Manage J 1995;38(5):1442–65.

28. Avolio BJ, Zhu W, Koh W, et al. Transformational leadership and organizational commitment: Mediating role of psychological empowerment and moderating role of structural distance. J Organizational Behav 2004;25(8):951–68.

29. Burns JM. Leadership. New York: Harper and Row; 1978.

30. Boamah SA, Spence Laschinger HK, Wong C, et al. Effect of transformational leadership on job satisfaction and patient safety outcomes. Nurs Outlook 2018; 66(2):180–9.

31. Afsar B, Umrani WA. Does thriving and trust in the leader explain the link between transformational leadership and innovative work behavior? A cross sectional survey. J Res Nurs 2020;25(1):37–51.

32. Khan BP, Griffin MTQ, Fitzpatrick JJ. Staff nurse's perceptions of their nurse managers transformational leadership behaviors and their own structural empowerment. J Nurs Adm 2018;48(12):609–14.

33. Specchia ML, Cozzolino MR, Carini E, et al. Leadership styles and nurses' job satisfaction: results of a systematic review. Int J Environ Res Public Health 2021;18:1552.

34. Madathil R, Heck NC, Schuldberg D. Burnout in psychiatric nursing: examining the interplay of autonomy, leadership style, and depressive symptoms. Arch Psychiatr Nurs 2014;28(3):160–6.

35. Lewis HS, Cunningham CJL. Linking nurse leadership and work characteristics to nurse burnout and engagement. Nurs Res 2016;65(1):13–23.

36. Cheng C, Bartram T, Karimi L, et al. Transformational leadership and social identity as predictors of team climate, perceived quality of care, burnout and turnover intention among nurses. Personnel Rev 2016;45(6):1200–16.

37. Boyatzis R, McKee A. Inspiring others through resonant leadership. Business Strategy Rev 2006;17(2):15–9.

38. Goleman D, Boyatzis R, McKee A. Review of primal leadership: realizing the power of emotional intelligence. Personnel Psychol 2002;55(4):1030–3.

39. Bawafaa E, Wong CA, Laschinger H. The influence of resonant leadership on the structural empowerment and job satisfaction of registered nurses. J Res Nurs 2015;20(7):610–22.

40. Laschinger HKS, Wong CA, Cummings GG, et al. Resonant leadership and workplace empowerment: The value of positive organizational cultures in reducing workplace incivility. Nurs Econ 2014;32(1):5–15.

41. Walumbwa FO, Avolio BJ, Gardner WL, et al. Authentic leadership: Development and Validation of a theory-based measure? J Management 2008;34:89–126.

42. Kim T-W, You Y-Y, Hong J-W. A study on the relationship among Servant Leadership, Authentic Leadership, Perceived Organizational Support(POS), and Agile Culture using PLS-SEM: Mediating Effect of POS. Ilkogretim Online 2021;20(3): 784–95.

43. Yousaf A, Ul Hadi N. Effect of psychological empowerment on authentic leadership and affective commitment relationship. J Managerial Sci 2020;14:109–98. Available at: https://search-ebscohost-com.ezp.waldenulibrary.org/login.aspx? direct=true&db=bth&AN=148243915&site=eds-live&scope=site.

44. Kotze M, Nel P. Personal factor effects on authentic leadership. J Psychol Africa 2017;27(1):47–53.

45. Laschinger HKS, Read EA. The effect of authentic leadership, person-job fit, and civility norms on new graduate nurses' experiences of coworker incivility and burnout. J Nurs Adm 2016;46(11):574–80.

46. Laschinger HKS, Wong CA, Grau AL. The influence of authentic leadership on newly graduated nurses' experiences of workplace bullying, burnout and retention outcomes: a cross-sectional study. Int J Nurs Stud 2012;49(10):1266–76.

47. Laschinger HKS, Fida R. A time-lagged analysis of the effect of authentic leadership on workplace bullying, burnout, and occupational turnover intentions. Eur J Work Organ Psychol 2014;23(5):739–53.

48. Laschinger HKS, Borgogni L, Consiglio C, et al. The effects of authentic leadership, six areas of worklife, and occupational coping self-efficacy on new graduate nurses' burnout and mental health: a cross-sectional study. Int J Nurs Stud 2015; 52(6):1080–9.

49. Boamah SA, Read EA, Laschinger HKS. Factors influencing new graduate nurse burnout development, job satisfaction and patient care quality: a time-lagged study. J Adv Nurs 2017;73(5):1182–95.

50. Rosseter R. Fact sheet: nursing shortage 2020. Available at: http://www.aacnnursing.org/News-Information/Fact-Sheets/Nursing-Shortage. Accessed June 29, 2021.

51. Wei H, King A, Jiang Y, et al. The impact of nurse leadership styles on nurse burnout: a systematic literature review. Nurs Leader 2020;18(5):439–50.

52. Gensimore MM, Maduro RS, Morgan MK, et al. The effect of nurse practice environment on retention and quality of care via burnout, work characteristics, and resilience: a moderated mediation model. JONA 2020;50:546–53.

Developing Resilience

Strategies to Adapt Within an Interprofessional Team

Victoria Hughes, DSN, MSN, RN[a],*,
Mary A. Bemker, PhD, PsyS, CNE, RN[b], Lynn C. Parsons, PhD, RN, NEA-BC[c]

KEYWORDS

• Resilience • Coping strategies • Adaptation • Interprofessional team

KEY POINTS

• Resilience is an important factor in addressing work stress, burnout, and turnover.
• Internal and external factors are important to build resilience.
• Strategies to promote resilience may include a mixture of supportive relationships, gratitude, meaningful recognition, and formal education programs.
• Strategies to promote highly effective teams may also affect team resilience.

INTRODUCTION

Nursing is one of the most demanding occupations across all types of work settings due to the physical, mental, and emotional demands that are placed on profession.[1] Findings from the American Nurses Association (2017) Health Risk Assessment revealed that 68% of nurses surveyed put the safety, wellness, and health of their patients before their own.[2] Nurses often worked through their breaks, experienced high levels of stress, and got less than recommended rest.[2] It is not surprising that in 2019, 15.6% of nurses within a national survey reported feelings of burnout.[3] In addition, the COVID-19 pandemic has increased both the patient care burden placed on nurses and the number of nurses that are experiencing burnout.[4] Health care organizations indicate that staff burnout is a patient safety and quality concern that needs to be quickly addressed.[5] Greater resilience demonstrated a protective effect on the burnout dimension of emotional exhaustion and contributed to personal accomplishment for 114 nurses working in high-intensity, stressful nursing settings.[6] According to a Joint Commission report, resilience is "the process of personal protection from burnout."[7]

[a] Johns Hopkins School of Nursing, 525 North Wolfe Street, Baltimore, MD 21205-2110, USA;
[b] College of Nursing, Graduate Program, Walden University, 100 Washington Avenue South, Suite 1210, Minneapolis, MN 55401, USA; [c] Department of Nursing, Morehead State University, School of Health Sciences, 101 Village Drive, Morehead, KY 40351, USA
* Corresponding author.
E-mail address: vhughes@jhu.edu

Nurs Clin N Am 57 (2022) 143–152
https://doi.org/10.1016/j.cnur.2021.11.010
0029-6465/22/© 2021 Elsevier Inc. All rights reserved.
nursing.theclinics.com

RESILIENCE DEFINITIONS

Resilience may be viewed as a trait, process, or even an outcome.[8] Resilience encompasses applications in biological, psychological, social, trauma, and moral/ethical domains but is not universally defined or applied.[9] There are multiple aspects of resilience, such as physical,[10] psychological,[11] moral,[12] and social.[13] Resilience may be conceptualized as a dynamic and multilevel phenomenon that may be examined at the individual, family, and community level.[14] For example, the interdependence of human biology (cellular, physiologic, and emotional) with expanding spheres of interactions with family, community, and society is one way to describe the complexity of resilience.[15]

Resilience exists along a developmental continuum[13] but may change over time in response to different types of stressors and contexts.[16] A unique aspect of resilience is that it manifests in a positive way during adverse life situations that typically lead to maladjustment.[17] Therefore, resilience is the capability of individuals, families, teams, or communities to cope with difficult situations by rebounding and adapt positively in response to the stressor.[18] In addition, resilience involves harnessing resources (internal and/or external) to sustain well-being when dealing with a perceived adversity.[19]

DISCUSSION
Resilience in Health Care

One strategy used for safety management in health care is resilience engineering. Resilience engineering adapts a safety approach to the constantly changing health care system's capacity to cope with complexity and variable conditions.[20] Resilient health care focuses on the factors and methods that enable individuals, teams, units, or the organization to adapt and cope effectively in everyday clinical work and different situations. Seven effective resilient health care factors identified in the literature include effective teamwork, in-situ practical experiences, exposure to diverse views and perspectives, using protocols, checklists, and a systems design, and team trade-offs and workarounds.[20]

Resilience Among Health Care Workers

Health care providers are the frontlines of emergencies and employment-related stress. High levels of injurious mental health consequences have been noted as a result.[21] Challenges generated by taxing clinical experiences, organizational culture and needs, and external factors that can affect an organization and the professionals within it (eg, lack of available personal protective equipments [PPEs]) are all variables associated with stress in health care settings.[22,23] Depending on the level of direct interaction, professional experience, and added stressors, dynamics linked to coping strategies are similar across health care professions. When high levels of stress and violence are not addressed properly in professional environs, health care providers may believe they are undervalued,[24] a key factor in burnout.[25,26]

Adaptations related to change and taxing events necessitates both physical and mental resilience. Resilience is defined as the ability to face difficult situations while simultaneously remaining focused and optimistic in a complicated health care environment.[27] Being able to evaluate resiliency promotes more effective preparation for resource allotment and development of interventions to support the health and well-being of individuals and organizations.[28] Further, this dynamic promotes the ability of both professionals and organizations to adapt functionality before, during, and after major events. The result is developing support for the necessary practices under expected and unexpected dynamics.[20]

The American Psychological Association (APA) identifies several factors associated with resilience regardless of profession.[29] The major variable identified to promote resiliency is positive and supportive relationships within and outside of the family unit. These relationships are believed to promote trust, acceptance, and encouragement. In addition, the APA notes that the ability to create and implement realistic plans, having a positive self-image, communication, and problem-solving skills, and the ability to govern emotions are also factors that support health and well-being. Both work environment and personal factors are associated with professional resiliency.

- Personal control within the health care environment seems to be a major source of resiliency. Without such, individual stressors are escalated in the health care setting.[22,30,31]
- Physical activity,[32] family support[30], leisure activity,[31] optimism, organizational tolerance skills, performing as a team member, maintaining professional boundaries, and maintaining a sense of humor were also noted as key variables among resilient professionals.[33]

Team Resilience

Factors that affect team performance may also affect team resilience. Findings from a qualitative study of health care team leaders and managers indicate that the team structure can facilitate team learning in resilience. When members experience their team as a helpful place to find solutions, model positive behaviors, and find ways to move forward during difficult situations, the team can be a very important vehicle for building and sustaining resilience. The perceived strength of the team relationships may not only affect the team effectiveness and performance but may also positively affect team learning and building resilience for dealing with adversity.[34]

Compassion, Presence, and Resilience Training (CPR-T) is a mindfulness-based and team-based intervention that uses a range of mindfulness practices and facilitator-led discussions with the oncology interprofessional teams.[35] CPR-T is designed to cultivate compassion, responsiveness, and self-care; strengthen presence, focused attention and calm, nonjudgmental acceptance; and build resilience, stamina, balance, and ability to face stressful circumstances. In a qualitative study of 10 CPR-T participants, 2 challenges and 5 benefits were identified. The 2 challenges involved committing to a sitting meditation practice and sharing vulnerability within the interprofessional teams. The participants were concerned that displaying vulnerability would be perceived negatively by group members who had a power differential. The benefits from attending the program included building self-compassion, receiving organization acknowledgment of stress, learning to pause, becoming fully present, and developing a working definition of stress and self-care. The participants described more empathy and presence in their interactions with patients and team members.[35]

Degbey and Einola discovered 3 specific underlying mechanisms, regulating emotions, self-reflection, and inclusion, that helped to cultivate team resilience.[36] Regulating and leveraging emotional expression by suppressing spontaneous negative emotions allowed participants to reflect and ultimately led to actions that promoted team inclusion. When teams invest resources in resilience building, they minimize the adversity impact by preparing for it, engaging in early detection, making sense of it, and selecting the most appropriate action to recover. Reflective practice is the key link between sensemaking and actions that promote resilience.[36] "Sensemaking involves turning circumstances into a situation that is comprehended explicitly in words and that serves as a springboard into action."[36] Sensemaking is portrayed as intertwined meaning and action.[37] Reflective practice is the process through which the sensemaking can occur.

STAFF NURSE RESILIENCE

Staff nurses face many challenges in the health care workforce. They comprise the greatest number of care providers while simultaneously practicing under difficult conditions. The saying *doing more with less* has taken on a different meaning in the current health care environment. The worldwide *coronavirus pandemic* (COVID-19) affected care delivery in all health care organizations in the United States and around the world.

Delivering high-quality care mandates intact leader capabilities to maintain a healthy, strong nursing workforce despite the challenges currently encountered: escalating costs; limited supplies, especially PPE; scarce nursing resources; and burnout among the nursing ranks.[27] Some of these challenges are listed as follows:

- High nurse turnover rates
- Costs associated with orienting new nurses
- Maintaining patient care quality
- Nurse stress and burnout
- Financial reimbursement from federal and health insurance agencies

---

Box 1
Resilience building strategies for staff nurses

1. *Facilitating Social Connections*—promoting social interactions in the workplace contributes to healthy interpersonal relations and builds a positive culture on different patient care units and the health care organization.

2. *Promoting Positivity*—being positive at work promotes an encouraging workplace. Use evidence-based approaches such as "Three Good Things," "Paying it Forward," and "Practicing Gratitude" promotes being positive at work and improves nurse resiliency.

3. *Capitalizing on Nurses' Strengths*—recognize individual strengths and use them to promote harmony and morale. By using the unique skill set of each nurse their self-confidence and work engagement increase.

4. *Nurturing Nurses' Growth*—involvement in nurse mentor programs facilitates the personal and professional development. Get the frontline nurses involved in committees and have them share what they are doing at nursing roundtables or lunches. An *open-door* policy with the nurse leader/manager facilitates *connections* between the staff nurse and their leader.

5. *Encouraging Nurses' Self-Care*—taking the time for self-care is important to maintain a healthy work-life balance. Nurse leaders can promote this through having restful break rooms off the main patient care unit and flexible scheduling. Adequate sleep, a healthy diet, and engaging in regular exercise are foundations of self-care.

6. *Fostering Mindfulness*—taking time to focus on the *moment* and closing out the past and future. Mindfulness reflects that the person is in the present and is fully engaged through active listening.

7. *Conveying Altruism*—a nurse leader conveys altruism by engaging in caring acts toward staff nurses with expecting anything in return. One of the easiest ways to convey a caring attitude toward others is to listen intently when others are speaking. Recognizing the good works of others conveys that their work is noticed and appreciated. Building nurse resilience can improve care delivery.

Data from Wei H, Roberts P, Strickler J, Corbett RW. Nurse leaders' strategies to foster nurse resilience. Journal of Nursing Management. 2019;27(4):681-687. doi:10.1111/jonm.12736.

Building Resiliency for Staff Nurses

The Triple Aim to the Quadruple Aim model to enhance the well-being of health care professionals was adopted by the Institute of Hospital Improvements.[27,38] Their trifold purpose is to reduce cost of care, advance population health, and enhance the practitioner's experience. Competing priorities make developing resilience strategies for nurses on the front lines of care delivery a vital skill to have in their repertoire.[39]

Nurse leaders must recognize issues that contribute to nurse burnout in the workplace so adverse outcomes can be minimized and interventions developed for healthy nurse coping.[40] Research completed by Wei and colleagues identified 7 resilience-building strategies for staff nurses.[27] The meaning of resilience building concepts are explained in **Box 1**.

Recognizing the contributions of staff nurses to the organization is an important component of the nurse manager role.[41] These investigators concluded that when the nurses' goals align with the organization's goals and values, a synergy is created that benefits the nurse and the organization. The nurse is recognized at the unit level and at the higher organizational level. Meaningful recognition within the organization builds individual capabilities and reinforces the organizations values, thereby establishing a strong, meaningful synergy. Resilient nurses are actively involved, compassionate, team oriented, and less likely to feel stressed, anxious, and burned out at work.[42]

Nurse Leader Role in Promoting Resiliency in Practice

A pilot program conducted at the University of Virginia studied resiliency and recognized that coping mechanisms that aided in stress reduction promoted job retention

Box 2	
Evidence-based strategies to promote positivity by nurse leaders	
Leader Strategy	**Description**
Three Good Things	Have staff nurses end their shift by sharing 3 good things that happened while at work.
	Nurse leaders start and end their meetings with 3 good things that happened to them during their day.
	Nurse executive encourages nurse managers, charge nurses, and nurse educators to begin their day using the "Three Good Things" strategy.
Practicing Gratitude	Encourage staff nurses to be grateful for the positive things that happened during their shift.
	Examples of this could be that she/he was able to call in the family in time to be at the bedside of their dying family member.
	A staff nurse shared that she was assigned a new nurse orientee to the unit and she was grateful for the extra pair of hands. The new nurse expressed gratitude for being mentored by a highly experienced expert clinician.
Paying it Forward	A Nurse Executive practices *paying it forward* after having a positive experience as a patient. The compassion inspired the leader to *pay it forward* to become a servant leader.
	An example of a Nurse Executive paying it forward is when the Chief Executive Officer (CEO) compliments her on decreased nursing division turnover at a cabinet meeting. The Nurse Executive *pays it forward* by recognizing publicly that the Critical Care Nurse Manager had zero sick time use during a busy year at the monthly manager meeting.

Data from Wei H, Roberts P, Strickler J, Corbett RW. Nurse leaders' strategies to foster nurse resilience. Journal of Nursing Management. 2019;27(4):681-687. doi:10.1111/jonm.12736.

> **Box 3**
> **A case profile for an advanced practice registered nurse**
>
> Case Profile
>   Dominica Sanchez, a nurse practitioner, has worked in health care for 25 years. She is starting
>   to feel sluggish and is having difficulty separating her work life with her personal life.
>   What kinds of things might Dominica want to consider in relation to resiliency?
>   What is one thing Dominica might do to promote resiliency?
>   Will the same factors be useful for her husband Sam Chen, a physical therapist for the same
>   organization?

and increased morale at work.[43] From their work, the following recommendations were made:

- Resiliency skill-building programs for middle managers by trained professionals
- Web-based resiliency courses for professional levels within the organization
- Dedicate time for nurse leader peer-to-peer connections and dedicate time to focus on well-being to support nurse leader resilience

Charge nurses, nurse executives, nurse middle managers, and nurse educators are in leader positions that can promote resiliency of frontline practitioners. There are many strategies that leaders can use to benefit nurses and the organization. Leading by example and being positive in the workplace affect nurse resiliency. Nurse leaders have used 3 evidence-based strategies that promote positivity: *Three Good Things*, *Practicing Gratitude*, and *Paying it Forward*.[27] The reader is referred to **Box 2** for the meaning of these strategies.

Resilience in Practice

When looking at conditions associated with overcoming, and even thriving during stressful times, it is imperative that direction is not limited entirely to lessening adversity and distress but also on increasing joy. Rippstein-Leuenberger and colleagues (2017) explore the content of health care practitioners—including nurses, physicians, and nurse practitioners—to the questions linked to 3 *"good things"* that happened that day and their part in making these events occur. Themes drawn from this investigation included *having a good day at work*, (2) *having supportive relationships*, and (3) *making meaningful use of self-determined time* (p.1).[44]

Resilience allows the health care professional to cope with work demands (volume, magnitude, and control of workload) supported by environmental factors within and outside of the workforce. Having these supports promotes professional performance and supports adjusting to change while continuing a sense of professional and personal gratification. Among primary care providers, character traits associated with high levels of self-determination and persistence are noted.[22] To further explore resilience in practice, please read the case profile and discuss the questions in **Box 3**.

SUMMARY

Nursing, as one of the most demanding occupations across all work types, places employees at a higher risk for stress, burnout, and high turnover rates. Burnout can negatively affect patient safety and quality. Resilience may help mitigate some of the negative outcomes related to demanding work environments. Personal factors such as physical activity,[32] leisure activity,[31] optimism, maintaining professional boundaries, and a sense of humor are associated with resilient professionals.[33] Environmental factors such as formal education, meaningful recognition, and social support[29] are potential building blocks for resilient nurses to remain focused and optimistic in the face of competing priorities and challenges in the constantly changing health care environment.[34] Resilience building programs are in alignment with the Quadruple Aim model designed to enhance the well-being of health care professionals. Programs such as the CPR-T, a mindfulness-based and team-based program, helps employees build self-compassion, receive organization acknowledgment of stress, learn to pause, become fully present, and develop a working definition of stress and self-care.[35] Furthermore, nurse leaders can foster resilience by facilitating social connections, promoting positivity, capitalizing on nurses' strengths, nurturing nurses' growth, encouraging nurses' self-care, fostering mindfulness practice, and conveying altruism. Recognizing the positive through *Three Good Things*, *Practicing Gratitude*, and *Paying it Forward* promotes an optimistic outlook, positive relationship, and resilience.[27] Resilience allows health care professionals to cope with challenging work demands, effectively adjust to change, and maintain a sense of meaning and personal gratification.

CLINICS CARE POINTS

- Resilience involves harnessing resources (internal and/or external) to sustain well-being. Internal nurse resources may include humor, professional boundaries, and physical/leisure activities.

- Formal education, meaningful recognition, and social support are building blocks for resilient nurses. Regulating emotions, self-reflection, and inclusion helps to cultivate team resilience.

- Practicing gratitude can positively affect relationships, sense of optimism, and nurse resilience.

- Health professional resilience may decrease the negative impact of demanding work environments and promote retention.

DISCLOSURE

None of the authors have any relationship with a commercial company that has a direct financial interest in subject matter or materials discussed in article or with a company making a competing product. The authors have nothing to disclose.

REFERENCES

1. American Association of Colleges of Nursing (AACN). Hallmarks of the professional nursing practice environment. J Prof Nurs 2002;18(5):295–304.
2. American Nurses Association. American Nurses Association health risk appraisal. Nursing World Website. 2007. Available at: https://www.nursingworld.org/~4aeeeb/globalassets/practiceandpolicy/work-environment/health—safety/anahealthriskappraisalsummary_2013-2016.pdf. Accessed April 10, 2021
3. King C, Bradley LA. Trends and Implications with Nursing Engagement: PRC Custom Research National Nursing Engagement Resource. 2019. Available at: https://prccustomresearch.com/wp-content/uploads/2019/PRC_Nursing_Engagement_Report/PRC-NurseReport-Final-031819-Secure.pdf. Accessed April 30, 2021.
4. Ross J. The exacerbation of burnout during covid-19: A major concern for nurse safety. J Perianesth Nurs 2020;35(4):439–40.
5. Annual patient safety & quality Industry outlook (2019). Kennesaw (GA): Patient Safety & Quality Healthcare (PSQH). 2019. Available at: psqh.com/intelligence. Accessed April 15, 2021.

6. Rushton CH, Batcheller J, Schroeder K, et al. Burnout and resilience among nurses practicing in high-intensity settings. Healthy Work Environments 2015; 24(5):412–20.

7. The Joint Commission. Quick Safety 50: Developing resilience to combat nurse burnout. 2019. Available at: https://bit.ly/2LEfcDc. Accessed April 15, 2021.

8. Reyes AT, Andrusyszyn M, Iwasiw C, et al. Nursing students' understanding and enactment of resilience: a grounded theory study. JAN 2015;71(11):2622–33. Available at: https://doi-org.proxy1.library.jhu.edu/10.1111/jan.12730.

9. Aburn G, Gott M, Hoare K. What is resilience? An integrative review of the empirical literature. JAN 2016;72:980–1000. https://doi.org/10.1111/jan.12888.

10. Whitson HE, Duan-Porter W, Schmader KE, et al. Physical resilience in older adults: Systematic review and development of an emerging construct. J Gerontol A Biol Sci Med Sci 2016;71(4):489–95.

11. Bartone PT. Resilience under military operational stress: can leaders influence hardiness? Mil Psychol 2006;18(Supplement):S131–48. https://doi.org/10.1207/s15327876mp1803s_10.

12. Holtz H, Heinze K, Rushton C. Interprofessionals' definitions of moral resilience. JCN 2018;27(3–4):e488–3494.

13. Bolzan N, Gale F. Using an interrupted space to explore social resilience with marginalized young people. Qual Soc Work 2011;11(5):502–16. https://doi-org.proxy1.library.jhu.edu/10.1177/1473325011403959.

14. Gucciardi DF, Crane M, Ntoumanis N, et al. J Occup Organ Psychol 2018;91(4): 729–68, 40p.

15. Szanton SL, Gill JM. (2010). Facilitating resilience using a society-to-cells framework: a theory of nursing essentials applied to research and practice. Adv Nurs Sci 2010;33(4):329–43.

16. Southwick SM, Bonanno GA, Masten AS, et al. Resilience definitions, theory, and challenges: interdisciplinary perspectives. Eur J Psychotraumatol 2014;5(1):1–14.

17. Luthar SS. Resilience in development: A synthesis of research across five decades. In: Cicchetti D, Cohen DJ, editors. Developmental psychopathology: risk, disorder, and adaptation. Hoboken, NJ: John Wiley & Sons, Inc.; 2006. p. 739–95.

18. Brennan EJ. Toward resilience and wellbeing in nurses. Br J Nurs 2017; 26(1):43–7.

19. Panter-Brick C, Leckman JF. Editorial Commentary: Resilience in child development – interconnected pathways to wellbeing. J Child Psychol Psychiatry 2013; 54(4):333–6.

20. Isflaifel M, Lim RH, Ryan K, et al. Resilient health care: A systematic review of conceptualizations, study methods and factors that develop resilience. BMC Health Serv Res 2020;(324):20. https://doi.org/10.1186/s12913-020-05208-3.

21. Wood AE, Prins A, Bush NE, et al. Reduction of burnout in mental health care providers using the provider resilience mobile application. Community Ment Health J 2017;53:452–9.

22. Robertson HD, Elliott AM, Burton CB, et al. Resilience of primary healthcare professionals: A systematic review. Br J Gen Pract 2016;66(647):e423–33.

23. Stephens TM, Smith P, Cherry C. Promoting resilience in new perioperative nurses. AORN J 2017;105:276–84.

24. Cherniack M. The productivity dilemma in workplace health promotion. Sci World J 2015. https://doi.org/10.1155/2015/937063. Article 937063.

25. Sidhu R, Su B, Shapiro KR, et al. Prevalence of and factors associated with burnout in midwifery: A scoping review. Eur J Midwifery 2020;4. https://doi.org/10.18332/ejm/115983.

26. Tang L, Pang Y, Chen Z, et al. Burnout among early-career oncology professionals and the risk factors. Psychooncology 2018;27(10):2436–41. https://doi.org/10.1002/pon.4847.

27. Wei H, Roberts P, Strickler J, et al. Nurse leaders' strategies to foster nurse resilience. J Nurs Manag 2019;27(4):681–7.

28. Barzilay R, Moore TM, Greenberg DM, et al. Resilience, COVID-19-related stress, anxiety and depression during the pandemic in a large population enriched for healthcare providers. Transl Psychiatry 2020;10:1–8. https://doi.org/10.1038/s41398-020-00982-4.

29. American Psychological Association. The road to resilience. Author. 2013. Available at: www.apa.org/helpcenter/road-resilience.aspx. Accessed April 1, 2021.

30. Bowden GE, Smith JC, Parker PA, et al. Working on the edge: Stresses and rewards of work in aa front-line mental health service. Clin Psychol Psychother 2015;22(6):488–501.

31. Zwack J, Schweitzer J. If every fifth physician is affected by burnout, what about the other four? Acad Med 2013;88(3):382–9.

32. Gerber M, Jonsdottir IH, Lindwall M, et al. Physical activity in employees with differing occupational stress and mental health profiles: A latent profile analysis. Psychol Sport Exerc 2014;15(6):649–58. https://doi.org/10.1016/j.psychsport.2014.07.012.

33. Mattheson C, Robertson HD, Elliott AM, et al. Resilience of primary healthcare professionals working in challenging environments: A focus group study. Br J Gen Pract 2016;648:e507–15. https://doi.org/10.3399/bjgp16X685285.

34. McCray J, Palmer A, Chmiel N. Building resilience in health and social care teams. Pers Rev 2016;45(6):1132–55.

35. Nissim R, Malfitano C, Coleman M, et al. A qualitative study of a compassion, presence, and resilience training for oncology interprofessional teams. J Holist Nurs 2019;37(1):30–44. https://doorg.proxy1.library.jhu.edu/10.1177/0898010118765016.

36. Degbey WY, Einola K. Resilience in virtual teams: Developing the capacity to bounce back. Appl Psychol Int Rev 2019;69(4):1301–37.

37. Weick KE, Sutcliffe KM, Obstfeld D. Organizing and the process of sensemaking. Organ Sci 2005;16(4):409–21. https://doi.org/10.1287/orsc.1050.0133.

38. Stiefel M, Nolan K. A guide to measuring the triple aim: Population health, experience of care, and per capita cost. Institute for healthcare improvement. 2012. Available at: http://www.ihi.org/resources/Pages/IHIWhitePapers/AGuidetoMeasuringTripleAim.aspx. Accessed April 18, 2021.

39. Kester K, Wei H. Building nurse resilience. Nurs Manag 2018;49(6):42–5. https://doi.org/10.1097/01.

40. Keyko K, Cummins G, Yonge O, et al. Work engagement in professional nursing practice: A systematic review. Int J Nurs Stud 2016;61:142–64.

41. Eddy JR, Kovick L, Caboral-Stevend M. Meaningful recognition: A synergy between the individual and the organization. Nurs Manag 2021;51(1):14–21.

42. Turner SB, Kaylor SD. Neuman Systems Model as a Conceptual Framework for Nurse Resilience. Nurs Sci Q 2015;28:213–7. https://doi.org/10.1177/0894318415585620.

43. Grim T, Delong A, Argenbright C. Trainable skills of wellbeing: A nurse manager resilience building pilot. University of Virginia. 2021. Available at: https://cdn. ymaws.com/virginianurses.com/resource/resmgr/exhibitor_details/Trainable_ Skills_of_Well-Bei.pdf. Accessed on April 10, 2021.
44. Rippstein-Leuenberger K, Mauthner O, Bryan Sexton J, et al. qualitative analysis of the Three Good Things intervention in healthcare workers. BMJ Open 2017;7: e015826.

Nursing Burnout and Its Impact on Health

Virginia Sullivan, MA[a],*, Vickie Hughes, DNS, MA, RN, CENP[b],
Debra Rose Wilson, PhD, MSN, RN, IBCLC, AHN-BC, CHT[c]

KEYWORDS

- Health • Burnout • Stress management • Self-care • Stress • Resilience

KEY POINTS

- Burnout is high in nursing and can have negative consequences for the mental and physical health of the nurse, as well as the organizational health of the hospital and the health of the patient.
- Burnout is a chronic stressor that results in reduced function of immune, cardiovascular, neuroendocrine, and central nervous systems.
- Self-care strategies and resilience promotion are needed to reduce burnout in nurses and improve health.

INTRODUCTION

Extensive demands are often placed on nurses in their workplace that can lead to high rates of burnout. Nurse burnout can have a vast array of negative consequences for the patient, the health care organization, the nursing profession, and the mental and physical health of the nurse as an individual. There are 3 primary health outcomes of burnout[1]: organizational health, mental health, and physical health.[1] Organizational health is the most widely researched of the three. It refers to organizational outcomes that occur when there are high rates of burnout within the organization, for example, lower quality of care, nurse retention, poor job performance, and so forth.[2] Mental health refers to the nurse's mental health as an individual, the high rates of trauma, depression, stress, and anxiety seen in many nurses, and how poor mental health often leads to burnout and vice-versa.[1] Poor physical health in nurses is often a result of high stress and burnout.[1] Burnout is conceptualized as a form of job stress. In this article, the authors discuss the relationship between stress and physical health and the toll that prolonged, increased stress can have on the body. The relationship between burnout and physical health is the least researched area within nursing burnout,

[a] Department of Pediatrics, Vanderbilt University Medical Center, 110 Magnolia Cir Room 407A, Nashville, TN 37203, USA; [b] School of Nursing, Johns Hopkins University, 525 North Wolfe Street, Baltimore, MD 21205, USA; [c] School of Nursing, Austin Peay State University, 1235 Jackson Cabin Road, Kingston Springs, TN 37211, USA
* Corresponding author.
E-mail address: ginger.sullivan@vumc.org

Nurs Clin N Am 57 (2022) 153–169
https://doi.org/10.1016/j.cnur.2021.11.011
0029-6465/22/© 2021 Elsevier Inc. All rights reserved.
nursing.theclinics.com

despite the fact that in 2001 one of the authors of the most widely used tools for measuring burnout (the Maslach Burnout Inventory [MBI]) called for more studies examining the physical health of health care workers, particularly nurses, as it relates to burnout as a facet of job stress.[1] The 3 facets of burnout and health are inextricably linked and will be discussed in relation to each other in this article. They also discuss findings and implications for each of these 3 facets of burnout and health in nursing.

BURNOUT INCIDENCE IN THE CONTEXT OF NURSING

Nurse burnout is a worldwide phenomenon negatively affecting patient safety, quality of patient care, health care professional health, and nurse retention.[2] According to a national nursing survey, 15.6% of more than 2000 nurses self-reported burnout.[3] Burnout in nursing is generally thought to be composed of 3 dimensions: emotional exhaustion (EE), depersonalization (DP), and reduced personal accomplishment (PA).[4] Emotional exhaustion is the state of exhaustion that stems from constant work in demanding conditions.[2] Depersonalization is the sensation of being detached from the care and treatment of patients.[2] Reduced personal accomplishment is the reduced sense of achievement experienced as a result of overworking and increased demands.[2]

The leading measurement on burnout, the MBI, assesses burnout based on these 3 dimensions of emotional exhaustion, depersonalization, and personal accomplishment.[5] The MBI is considered the "gold standard" for assessing burnout, particularly in health professions. It is widely used in studies examining professional burnout and shows strong validity in several populations and languages.[6]

Symptoms of burnout can be classified into 4 main categories: emotional, cognitive, behavioral, and social symptoms.[4] Examples of emotional symptoms are hopelessness, apathy, depression, helplessness, and irritation. Some cognitive symptoms may be cognitive disorientation, distraction, loss of meaning, and loss of value. Behavioral symptoms involve maladaptive behavior such as increased consumption of substances, avoidance of responsibility, and absenteeism. Social symptoms often involve interpersonal conflicts, deteriorated relations at home, and social isolation.[4] Nurse burnout negatively affects registered nurse turnover rates, threatens patient safety, and results in poor job performance.[2] The Joint Commission (2019)[7] released a statement that health care organizations have a responsibility to support nurses and address the causes of nurse burnout.

RISK FACTORS FOR NURSE BURNOUT

Several factors may contribute to nurse burnout, such as workload, moral distress, flawed support system, limited resources, limited training, and bullying.[8] In addition, anxiety, depression, physical and mental exhaustion, and depersonalization may result as effects of prolonged exposure to stress, leading to nurse burnout.[8] Extended work hours, mandatory overtime, staff shortages, time constraints, poor management, low nurse-to-patient ratios, and a lack of team support have also been critical factors associated with registered nurse burnout.[2] In addition, witnessing a traumatic event at work such as an assault, working lengthy periods of primary shift work, and years of nursing practice may also influence the nurses' risk for burnout.[9] Working in practice areas with increased patient morbidity and mortality, ethical dilemmas, and physically and mentally demanding daily nursing practices, such as critical care and the emergency department, may place nurses at higher risk for burnout.[10] Increases in workplace violence and moral distress experiences in the emergency department have been associated with nurse burnout.[11] Furthermore, emergency department nurse burnout has been associated with nurse perception factors such as feeling unappreciated, excessive work volume, unable to meet job expectations, and lack of time to properly perform duties.[11]

PROTECTIVE FACTORS FOR NURSE BURNOUT

Protective factors for burnout in nurses working with patients admitted to a hospital following traumatic injury included being female, being married, and better quality of sleep.[9] As defined as the assistance and protection given by others, social support is a predictive and protective factor for nurse burnout.[4] Social support is also one of the attributes of resilience.[12] Additional attributes of resilience that may be protective include rebounding, coping or adapting, self-determination, and a positive outlook.[12]

Resilience can be viewed as a trait, process, or outcome depending on the specified context.[13] A unique aspect of resilience is that it manifests during negative life situations that typically lead to maladjustment but promotes a positive adaptation.[14] Resilience involves a developmental progression that changes over time with new vulnerabilities and strengths emerging in response to changing life circumstances.[14] Different dimensions (physical, emotional, social, moral, or psychological) of resilience may manifest during a response to adversity.[15] According to a Joint Commission report, resilience is "the process of personal protection from burnout."[7]

Resilience, hope, and support were found to reduce emotional exhaustion in 114 nurses who worked in high-stress nursing units.[16] Greater resilience demonstrated a protected effect, for nurses working in high-intensity settings, on the burnout dimension of emotional exhaustion and contributed to personal accomplishment.[16] Spiritual well-being was noted to reduce emotional exhaustion and depersonalization.[16]

HEALTH CONSEQUENCES OF BURNOUT

It has long been known that chronic stress has adverse effects on physical and emotional health. Burnout is a chronic stressor that results in reduced function of immune, cardiovascular, neuroendocrine, and central nervous systems. The longer the stress is perceived, the more the immune system responds. Eventually, cellular immunity is exhausted, and the cytokine call for inflammation in the body is triggered. Nonessential immune functions are shut down, and this might include stopping the development of natural killer cells whose job is to kill mutating cancer cells before they get out of hand.[17] Not only is normal immune system function disrupted (opening the door for illness), but stress-triggered inflammation leads to other problems. Metabolic syndrome has an underlying factor of inflammation and then contributes to the formation of cardiovascular disease, diabetes, hypertension, and stroke. Stress and burnout lead to inflammation. Disease develops. Irritable bowel syndrome (an inflammatory auto-immune disease) was directly associated with burnout, for example.[18] Burnout increases CVD risk as much as smoking or obesity.[19] CVD is triggered and escalated by inflammation and is in itself inflammatory. As stress increases, the anti-inflammatory cell production is reduced, and inflammation rages through the body.

Sleep deprivation is associated with burnout and has negative effects on health. Reduced sleep results in higher blood pressure and inflammation. Inadequate sleep is strongly linked to an increased risk of dying. Sleep deprivation increases inflammation and triggers the genesis or relapse of disease.[17] Quality sleep enhances immune defense.[20] Sleep deprivation–associated inflammation is a predictor of suicidal ideation.[21] There is also an effect on emotional and cognitive function with inadequate sleep.[22] Increased posttraumatic stress disorder (PTSD) diagnosis is not surprising after health care workers dealt with the COVID-19 pandemic and is an extreme part of the burnout continuum. Sleep disturbances and inflammation accompany PTSD and can be experienced by those with burnout.[23]

High scores on the MBI predicted future psychotropic drug use in an older longitudinal study.[24] One study found that 45% of those working on the frontline of COVID-19 surveyed reported at least one physical symptom in the last 4 weeks, many related to health issues with long-lasting consequences.[25]

Increased PTSD diagnosis is not surprising after health care workers dealt with the COVID-19 pandemic and is an extreme part of the burnout continuum. Sleep disturbances and inflammation accompany PTSD and can be experienced by those with burnout.[23]

There is a strong link between inflammation and depression (and other psychiatric illnesses). Depression is an inflammatory condition that worsens other inflammatory conditions in the body. Depression increases when inflammatory diseases (such as rheumatoid arthritis) are active.[17] The inflammatory factors of depression can predict the risk of cancer. Physicians who scored high on the Maslach had higher levels of alcohol abuse, depression, poor self-care, and motor vehicle crashes.[26]

Long-term and unremitting stress can reduce the function of the immune system even more. The continuous presence of stress hormones triggers more inflammation, which is a risk factor for ulcers, Alzheimer disease, and other autoimmune diseases.[17] The health of nurses and other health care practitioners is influenced by inflammation, and burnout contributes to poor health.

RESEARCH ON NURSE BURNOUT AND HEALTH

The MBI is the most widely used tool to measure burnout in nursing, and in this section, the authors focus on findings related to burnout and health using this validated tool.[6] There are 5 versions of the MBI (MBI-HSS for workers in human services, MBI-HSS [MP] for medical personnel specifically, MBI-ES for workers in educational settings, MBI-GS for workers in other occupational groups, and MBI-GS [S] for college and university students).[5] Most studies in this review used the MBI-HSS; however, a few used the MBI-GS. The MBI-HSS measures the 3 dimensions of burnout discussed earlier (emotional exhaustion, depersonalization, and personal achievement), whereas the MBI-GS measures 3 different dimensions (exhaustion, cynicism, and professional efficacy).[5] It should be noted here that some of the articles discussed in this section used this alternate version of the MBI.

In the systematic review by Zangaro and colleagues,[27] 2391 articles from the years 2000 to 2019 were first filtered for titles and abstracts that included the MBI and were written in English. To identify findings related to health, these 2391 articles were screened for health-related research findings in nurses. In this section, the authors report on findings and conclusions from these articles. Fourteen articles were identified that measured mental health or physical health either as outcomes of burnout or as alongside burnout. **Table 1** summarizes findings from these 14 articles. Unfortunately, very few articles correlated health with burnout. Most investigators chose to use burnout as a measure of stress or mental health alongside another scale measuring health and to compare both with other factors that may be contributing to overall mental health, such as poor work environment. These results are often combined to give a general idea of overall mental health, and it is difficult to decipher the relationship between burnout and health.

MENTAL HEALTH FINDINGS

Several different scales examined various aspects of mental health in the research in this review. As most researchers viewed burnout as a facet of job stress, stress was

Table 1
Burnout and mental- and physical health–related findings

Tool Used to Measure Health	Article Reference	Sample	Findings
Mental Health			
Perceived Stress Scale (PSS)[28]	Fernandez-Sanchez et al,[29] 2018	69 palliative health care workers (32 nursing assistants, 30 nurses, 7 physicians)[29]	Participants with high levels on one or more burnout dimensions showed higher average scores on the perceived stress scale.[29]
Symptoms Checklist-90 (SCL-90)[30]	Fernandez-Sanchez et al,[29] 2018	69 palliative health care workers (32 nursing assistants, 30 nurses, 7 physicians)[29]	Participants with high levels of burnout on at least one dimension also had higher levels of interpersonal sensitivity, depression, hostility, and paranoid ideation. They also showed higher scores on the global severity index and positive symptom total.[29]
	Qiao et al,[31] 2016	492 infectious disease health care workers (264 physicians and nurses caring for HIV/AIDS, 228 caring for other infectious diseases)[31]	Health care workers working in HIV/AIDS showed higher total scores on the SCL-90 compared with health care workers working with other infectious diseases. High psychoticism scores were associated with burnout.[31]
Secondary Traumatic Stress Scale (STSS)[32]	Favros et al,[33] 2018	122 midwives & 91 NICU nurses[33]	Secondary traumatic stress symptoms were above the threshold in 26.9% of midwives and 50% of NICU nurses. Both groups showed high levels of burnout.[33]

(continued on next page)

Table 1
(continued)

Tool Used to Measure Health	Article Reference	Sample	Findings
Hospital Anxiety and Depression Scale (HADS)[34]	Favros et al,[33] 2018	122 midwives & 91 NICU nurses[33]	Anxiety symptoms were significantly higher in midwives (19.3%) than NICU nurses (12%). Both groups showed high levels of burnout.[33]
	Mealer et al,[35] 2012	744 nurses[35]	Anxiety, depression, and burnout were common in ICU nurses. 18% were positive for symptoms of anxiety and 11% were positive for symptoms of depression. There was a high rate of burnout syndrome with 80% of nurses having positive symptoms in at least 1 of the 3 individual dimensions.[35]
10-item Connor-Davidson Resilience Scale[36]	Arrogante & Aparicio-Zaldivar,[37] 2017	52 critical care professionals (nurses, nursing assistants, and physicians)[37]	The 3 burnout dimensions were negatively associated with resilience. Resilience mediated the relationship between each of the 3 dimensions of burnout and mental health.[37]
	Mealer et al,[35] 2012	744 nurses[35]	All 3 dimensions of burnout were significantly lower in nurses who had high resilience.[35]
Short Form-12 Health Survey (SF-12)[38]	Arrogante & Aparicio-Zaldivar,[37] 2017	52 critical care professionals (nurses, nursing assistants, and physicians)[37]	Resilience reduced the impact of negative mental health consequences of burnout. Resilience partially mediated the relationship between emotional exhaustion and depersonalization with mental health and totally mediated the relationship between personal accomplishment and mental health.[37]

General Health Questionnaire-28 (GHQ-28)[39]	Khamisa et al,[40] 2016	277 nurses[40]	Burnout was significantly associated with poor general health, manifesting as headaches and depression.[40]
Symptoms Rating Scale for Depression and Anxiety (SRSDA)[41]	Papathanasiou,[42] 2015	240 health care workers (183 nurses, 25 physicians, 5 midwives, 16 other)[42]	The burnout dimensions of emotional exhaustion and personal accomplishment were associated (either positively or negatively) with depression, melancholia, asthenia, anxiety, and mania.[42]
General Health Questionnaire-12 (GHQ-12)[43]	Sacadura-Liete et al,[44] 2014	136 hospital nurses[44]	Stress and burnout were not discussed in relation to each other in this study. Stress was used as an independent variable to measure effectiveness of the influenza vaccine in nurses.[44]
Short Form-36 Health Survey (SF-36)[45]	Suner-Soler et al[46] 2013	1095 health care workers (nurses, physicians, nursing assistants, and orderlies)[46]	High levels of burnout, particularly the emotional exhaustion dimension, showed a deterioration in mental health.[46]
	Anagnostopoulos & Niakas,[47] 2010	487 nurses[47]	Personal accomplishment was positively and significantly associated with mental health. Those with short-term sickness absence had both low mental health scores and high burnout.[47]
Posttraumatic Diagnostic Scale (PDS)[48]	Mealer et al,[35] 2012	744 nurses[35]	Prevalence of PTSD in this sample was 21%, with 70% of those nurses showing symptoms for 3 mo. Resilience was associated with lower prevalence of PTSD. Post-traumatic stress was not correlated with burnout in this study.[35]

(continued on next page)

Table 1
(continued)

Tool Used to Measure Health	Article Reference	Sample	Findings
State–Trait Anxiety Inventory (STAI)[49]	Albini et al,[50] 2011	230 health care workers (physicians, nurses, and ancillary staff)[50]	The MBI and STAI were used together as measures of stressors and strain and were used in combination to analyze factors of job content.[50]
Pressure Management Indicator (PMI)[51]	Harwood et al,[52] 2010	121 nephrology nurses[52]	"For every standardized unit increase in emotional exhaustion and cynicism, mental health symptom scores decreased (worsened) by (−.353) and (−.333), respectively. Of the 2 measures of burnout examined, it was emotional exhaustion that had the greater impact on mental health symptoms. As the nurses experienced mental health symptoms such as feeling nervous, down in the dumps, not calm, downhearted and blue, and not happy, scores decreased."[52]
Physical Health			
Salivary cortisol testing	Fernandez-Sanchez et al,[29] 2018	69 palliative health care workers (32 nursing assistants, 30 nurses, 7 physicians)[29]	Those who showed burnout in at least one dimension had a higher release of cortisol on waking and at bedtime but had the same as their non-burned-out counterparts during the workday.[29]
Short Form-12 Health Survey (SF-12)[38]	Arrogante & Aparicio-Zaldivar,[37] 2017	52 critical care professionals (nurses, nursing assistants and physicians)[37]	The emotional exhaustion dimension of burnout was negatively associated with physical health.[37]

21-item scale asking participants to report the occurrence of health symptoms within the past year[53]	Skorobogatova et al,[53] 2017	94 neonatal intensive care nurses[53]	Tiredness was associated with burnout.[53]
Health Behavior Questionnaire[54]	Alexandrova-Karamanova et al,[54] 2017	2623 health care workers (1431 nurses, 627 physicians, 565 residents)[54]	Higher scores of emotional exhaustion and depersonalization were significantly associated with more frequent fast-food consumption, less frequent exercise, more frequent alcohol consumption, and more frequent painkiller use.[54]
Symptoms Checklist-90 (SCL-90)[30]	Fernandez-Sanchez et al,[29] 2018	69 palliative health care workers (32 nursing assistants, 30 nurses, 7 physicians)[29]	Participants with high levels of burnout on at least one dimension also had higher levels on the global severity index and the positive symptoms total.[29]
	Qiao et al,[31] 2016	492 infectious disease health care workers (264 physicians and nurses caring for HIV/AIDS, 228 caring for other infectious diseases)[31]	Burnout symptoms were significantly higher in HIV/AIDS health care workers who had serious somatization and poor quality of sleep.[31]
General Health Questionnaire-28 (GHQ-28)[39]	Khamisa et al,[40] 2016	277 nurses[40]	High levels of burnout were associated with general health, with emotional exhaustion being most significantly associated.[40]
General Health Questionnaire-12 (GHQ-12)[43]	Sacadura-Liete et al[44] 2014	136 hospital nurses[44]	Results from the MBI were not discussed in the results of this study, and burnout was not discussed in relation to physical health.[44]

(continued on next page)

Table 1
(continued)

Tool Used to Measure Health	Article Reference	Sample	Findings
Short Form-36 Health Survey (SF-36)[45]	Suner-Soler et al[46] 2013	1095 health care workers (nurses, physicians, nursing assistants, and orderlies)[46]	High levels of burnout, particularly emotional exhaustion, showed a deterioration in physical health. Depersonalization was associated more with mental health than physical health.[46]
	Anagnostolopoulos & Niakas[47] 2010	487 nurses[47]	The emotional exhaustion and depersonalization subscales were associated with physical health.[47]
Data on sick leaves from hospital personnel records	Anagnostolopoulos & Niakas[47] 2010	487 nurses[47]	Nurses with high levels of burnout were more likely to be absent from work for a short time than those with low levels of burnout.[47]
Pressure Management Indicator (PMI)[51]	Harwood et al[52] 2010	121 nephrology nurses[52]	Emotional exhaustion had a significant effect on physical symptoms (feeling tired or exhausted, short of breath, muscles trembling, prickling sensation).[52]

commonly examined, contributing to overall stress.[29,33,35,50] Fernandez-Sanchez and colleagues[29] directly correlated stress, as measured by the perceived stress scale, and burnout, finding that those with high levels of burnout on one or more of the 3 dimensions showed higher average scores on the perceived stress scale.[29] Posttraumatic stress was also measured by 2 of the studies.[33,35] Favros and colleagues[33] found that 50% of neonatal intensive care unit nurses experience secondary stress; these nurses also experienced high levels of burnout.[33] Mealer and colleagues[35] examined 744 nurses and found that 21% exhibited symptoms of PTSD, with 70% of those nurses experiencing symptoms for at least 3 months.[35] Mealer and colleagues[35] did not report whether or not nurses experiencing symptoms of PTSD were also burned out. However, they reported that 80% of nurses in their sample met the criteria for at least one of the burnout dimensions.[35]

The Mealer and colleagues'[35] study aimed to examine the role of resilience in nurses experiencing PTSD, burnout, anxiety, and depression. The investigators identify several exciting findings related to the mental health of nurses. They measured resilience using the 10-item Connor-Davidson Resilience Scale.[36] They tested for associations between resilience and each of the variables mentioned earlier, finding a significant association between resilience and lower prevalence of PTSD (8% prevalence in those who were highly resilient vs 25% in those who were not highly resilient, $P < .001$), lower burnout in all 3 dimensions ($P < .001$), and psychological symptoms (significantly lower prevalence of anxiety [8% vs 21%, $P = .001$] and depression [2% vs 14%, $P < .001$]),[35] meaning that more resilient nurses were more likely to report general satisfaction with their lives than less resilient nurses.[35]

Depression and anxiety were measured in several studies using the SCL-90,[30] the HADS,[34] the SF-12,[38] the GHQ-28,[39] the SRSDA,[41] the SF-36,[45] and the Pressure Management Indicator (PMI).[51] Some studies did not correlate burnout and depression, anxiety, or other mental health disorders measured by these instruments with burnout. Those who did correlate depression and anxiety with burnout found significant relationships between high burnout and poor mental health, especially symptoms of depression.[29,31,33,35,40,42,46,47,52] The investigators also reported other aspects of poor mental health in nurses with high burnout, including interpersonal sensitivity,[29] hostility,[29] paranoid ideation,[29] psychoticism,[31] melancholia,[42] asthenia,[42] mania,[42] feeling nervous,[52] down in the dumps,[52] not calm,[52] downhearted and blue,[52] and not happy.[52]

PHYSICAL HEALTH FINDINGS

As discussed earlier in this article, burnout is often conceptualized as job stress, contributing to poor mental health, and poor mental health can lead to inflammation and several adverse physical health illnesses. Many research studies examined mental and physical health side-by-side, presumably for this reason. Arrogante and Aparicio-Zaldivar[37] used the SF-12[38] in their study, asking participants questions about mental and physical health. The aim of their study was to examine the role of resilience in burnout and mental and physical health.[37] When comparing burnout and physical health, they found an association between emotional exhaustion and physical health.[37] Interestingly, when examining the role of resilience, they found that resilience mediated the relationship between all 3 dimensions of burnout and mental health (EE: $\beta = -0.38$, $P < .01$, DP: $\beta = -0.20$, $P < .01$, PA: $\beta = 0.07$, $P < .05$).[37] However, they did not find this moderation in physical health.[37] In fact, they did not find a relationship between resilience and physical health at all.[37]

Suner-Soler and colleagues[46] and Anagnostolopoulos and Niakas[47] also used a version of the short-form survey, SF-36,[45] to examine both mental and physical health.

Suner-Soler and colleagues[46] found a significant relationship between burnout and diminished physical health, with the emotional exhaustion scale showing a more substantial relationship than the other 2 dimensions.[46] They also found that the depersonalization scale had a stronger relationship with mental health than physical health, which was not true for emotional exhaustion and personal accomplishment.[46] Anagnostolopoulos and Niakas[47] identified a relationship between the emotional exhaustion and depersonalization dimensions and poor physical health.[47] Other scales used to measure mental and physical health were the SCL-90,[30] the GHQ-28,[39] the GHQ-12,[43] and the PMI.[51] The identified studies using these measures identify a relationship between burnout and poor physical health outcomes.[29,31,37,40,44,46,47,52-54] Some specific physical outcomes reported were somatization,[31] poor quality of sleep,[31] tiredness,[53] feeling tired or exhausted,[52] short of breath,[52] trembling muscles,[52] and prickling sensations.[52]

Some research focused on more specific aspects of physical health. In this review, research was found on salivary cortisol,[29] influenza vaccine efficacy,[44] risky health behaviors,[54] and time off for sick leave.[47] Fernandez-Sanchez and colleagues[29] examined salivary cortisol levels in health care workers (mostly nurses). They found that those who scored high in at least one dimension of burnout had higher salivary cortisol levels in the morning and around bedtime but similar levels as non–burned-out co-workers during the workday ($F(3.5) = 2.48$, $P < .03$).[29] This finding provides evidence that health care workers who are more burned out are experiencing more dysregulation of the hypothalamic-pituitary-adrenal (HPA) axis, which helps regulate homeostasis in the body during stressful situations.[29] Another research has found that workers with a regulated HPA-axis engage with their work to a greater extent.[29]

Sacadura-Liete and colleagues[44] examined the efficacy of the influenza vaccine in hospital nurses who were or not experiencing high levels of stress and burnout. Unfortunately, in the results of their article, they did not discuss their findings related to burnout, only chronic stress as measured by the GHQ-12.[43,44] They did, however, find that there was a drop in immune response (measured by hemagglutination inhibition antibodies) 6 months after vaccination in nurses who were experiencing high levels of chronic stress.[44]

Another study examined risky health behaviors in 2623 health care workers (1431 nurses) and found that higher emotional exhaustion and depersonalization were significantly associated with more frequent fast-food consumption (EE: $F = 44.18$, $P < .001$; DP: $F = 60.83$, $P < .001$), less frequent exercise (EE: $F = 70.64$, $P < .001$; DP: $F = 30.66$, $P < .001$), more frequent alcohol consumption (EE: $F = 8.40$, $P < .01$; DP: $F = 29.66$, $P < .001$), and more frequent painkiller use (EE: $F = 148.99$, $P < .001$; DP: $F = 74.91$, $P < .001$).[54] These risky health behaviors have negative consequences for the health of the individual nurse. Other studies have also found that engaging in these behaviors can lead to medical errors, inadequate patient safety, and health promotion directed toward patients.[54]

Anagnostolopoulos and Niakas[47] examined time-off for sick leave of 477 nurses. Increased sick leave affects both the individual nurse and the organization.[47] It could mean that those with increased sick leave are experiencing more illness, and the organization suffers when there is a higher rate of absence of nurses. They found that nurses with high levels of burnout were more likely to be absent from work for a short time than those with low levels of burnout.[47] The investigators recommend that hospitals implement programs to reduce absence and pay special attention to nurses with short-term sickness absences because this may be an indicator of someone who is burned out and may benefit from support from the hospital.[47]

DISCUSSION

There is a clear connection between burnout and health, and as health care professionals, nurses need to seek education to further embrace their self-care as a prevention and treatment method. Strategies for dealing with stressors of work, personal life, and a pandemic need to be intentionally sought out and practiced. Health care professionals who have had to deal with COVID-19 are under even more psychological strain with high rates of PTSD.[55] Burnout is easily monitored with validated surveys such as the MBI to recognize when preventive approaches were not enough. Treatment approaches are then required, coming from facilities, the individuals themselves, and the professional organizations. The American Nurses Association and the American Holistic Nurses Association have online free resources to assist health care professionals in becoming self-aware and applying self-care concepts.

Burnout was associated with several mental health symptoms, but stress, anxiety, and depression, in particular, showed strong relationships with burnout in several studies.[29,33,35,40,42,52] It was also found that mental health symptoms were more strongly associated with the emotional exhaustion domain than depersonalization or personal accomplishment in 2 studies.[46,52] Leaders in nursing would benefit from implementing programs that stress the importance of being mindful of personal mental health needs and emotional exhaustion and being attuned to the mental health needs of the nurses under their leadership. These programs include tools to help identify when they are becoming emotionally exhausted and help them access mental health counseling or therapy and techniques to promote self-care and mindfulness. A caring and supportive environment can go a long way in making nurses feel they can ask for help when they need it.

If mental health needs and burnout are not addressed, it can lead to adverse physical health outcomes. In the articles reviewed, the most commonly reported physical health outcome related to burnout was tiredness or poor quality of sleep.[31,52,53] As reported by Zangaro and colleagues, workload is a primary stressor contributing to burnout, and excessive workload may lead to a lack of a proper sleep schedule.[27] Increased workload is also correlated with emotional exhaustion, which can indirectly affect patient care.[27] Organizations and leaders in nursing can improve the health of nurses by decreasing the workload on nurses. The emotional exhaustion subscale was more strongly related to negative physical health outcomes than the other 2 subscales in several studies.[37,40,46,47,52,54] When nurses are emotionally exhausted it affects not only their personal mental and physical health but also patient care, job satisfaction, and nurse retention.[27,36,40,46,47,52,54] It is critical that organizations and leaders in nursing address emotional exhaustion and burnout in their nursing staff; this can be done through creating a supportive environment and implementing programs that foster a caring environment and promote a healthy work/life balance, including access to mental health counseling, promoting self-care, and mindfulness techniques.

Resilience seemed to have a mediating effect on the relationship between burnout and health in one study[37] and was associated with lower burnout scores in another.[35] Health care organizations that implement resilience training may reduce burnout rates, increase staff retention, and improve patient safety. However, the training will not produce the desired outcomes unless there is an environment of mutual trust, psychological safety, and empowerment.[56] Facilitating social connections, promoting positivity, capitalizing on nurses' strengths, nurturing nurses' growth, encouraging nurses' self-care, fostering mindfulness practice, and conveying altruism are strategies identified by nurse leaders to promote resilience.[57] Despite nurse executives' indication that resiliency promotion is a priority, the increase in violence at point-of-care, nurses' perception of the need to take short-cuts in patient care delivery, no time to recover from stressful and traumatic situations, and being alone due to care protocols contribute to nurses' feelings of isolation and undermine nurses' ability to improve resilience.[58]

SUMMARY

Nurse burnout and health are shown to be correlated by several studies examining both mental and physical health.[29,31,33,35,37,40,42,44,46,47,50,52–54] Nurse burnout also leads to poor organizational health through staff retention, patient safety, and increased short-term absence, among others.[2] Nurses who have burned out show signs of poor overall mental health,[37,46,47,52] depression,[29,35,40,42] anxiety,[33,35,42] and chronic stress,[29,33,35,44] when measured by multiple instruments. Chronic and posttraumatic stress has a significant toll on the body through metabolic syndrome and inflammation, leading to more severe diseases, such as cardiovascular disease, diabetes, hypertension, and stroke. The effects of burnout and stress on the physical health of nurses are also seen in several research studies. These studies examined physical health outcomes such as influenza vaccine immunity,[44] time off for sick days,[47] risky health behaviors,[54] and so forth. Resilience was examined in 2 studies and was found to have a positive impact on lowering burnout and its mental and physical outcomes and was even found to mediate the relationship between all 3 dimensions of burnout and mental health.[35,37] Self-care is an effective tool to lower chronic stress. The authors recommend that hospitals and organizations focus on programs that implement resilience training and promote self-care to combat burnout and its adverse effects on health.

CLINICS CARE POINTS

- Promote healthy lifestyles, including exercise and proper nutrition.
- Mental health support.
- Promoting self-care is imperative to provide quality care to patients.
- Implement resilience training in order to combat burnout and its negative effects on health.

DISCLOSURE

The authors have nothing to disclose.

REFERENCES

1. Maslach C. What have we learned about burnout and health? Psychol Health 2001;16(5):607–11.
2. Bakhamis L, Paul DP III, Smith H, et al. Still an epidemic: the burnout syndrome in hospital registered nurses. Health Care Manag 2019;38(1):3–10.
3. Brusie C. Study reveals alarming statistics on nurse burnout. 2019. Available at: https://nurse.org/articles/nurse-burnout-statistics/. Accessed July 8, 2021.
4. Gómez-Urquiza JL, Albendín-García L, Velando-Soriano A, et al. burnout in palliative care nurses, prevalence and risk factors: a systematic review with meta-analysis. Int J Environ Res Public Health 2020;17(20):7672.
5.. Maslach C, Jackson SE, Leiter MP. Maslach burnout inventory: third edition. In: Zalaquett CP, Wood RJ, editors. Evaluating stress: a book of resources. Lanham, MD: Scarecrow Education; 1997. p. 191–218.

6. Poghosyan L, Aiken LH, Sloane DM. Factor structure of the Maslach burnout inventory: an analysis of data from large scale cross-sectional surveys of nurses from eight countries. Int J Nurs Stud 2009;46(7):894–902.

7. The Joint Commission issues quick safety advisory on combating nurse burnout through resilience. 2019. Available at: https://www.jointcommission.org/resources/news-and-multimedia/news/2019/07/the-joint-commission-issues-quick-safety-advisory-on-combating-nurse-burnout-through-resilience/. Accessed July 8, 2021.

8. Brown S, Whichello R, Price S. The impact of resiliency on nurse burnout: An integrative literature review. Medsurg Nurs 2018;27(6):349.

9. Higgins JT, Okoli C, Otachi J, et al. Factors Associated With Burnout in Trauma Nurses. J Trauma Nurs 2020;27(6):319–26.

10. Browning SG. Burnout in critical care nurses. Crit Care Nurs Clin North Am 2019; 31(4):527–36.

11. Rozo JA, Olson DM, Thu H, et al. Situational factors associated with burnout among emergency department nurses. Workplace Health Saf 2017;65(6):262–5.

12. Caldeira S, Timmins F. Resilience: synthesis of concept analyses and contribution to nursing classifications. Int Nurs Rev 2016;63(2):191–9.

13. Reyes AT, Andrusyszyn MA, Iwasiw C, et al. Nursing students' understanding and enactment of resilience: a grounded theory study. J Adv Nurs 2015;71(11): 2622–33.

14. Luthar SS. Resilience in development: a synthesis of research across five decades. In: Cicchetti D, Cohen DJ, editors. Developmental psychopathology: risk, disorder, and adaptation. Hoboken, NJ: John Wiley & Sons, Inc.; 2006. p. 739–95.

15. Southwick SM, Bonanno GA, Masten AS, et al. Resilience definitions, theory, and challenges: interdisciplinary perspectives. Eur J Psychotraumatol 2014;5(1): 25338.

16. Rushton CH, Batcheller J, Schroeder K, et al. Burnout and resilience among nurses practicing in high-intensity settings. Am J Crit Care 2015;(5):412–20.

17. Wilson DR. Psychoneuroimmunology. In: Blaszko Helming MA, Shields DA, Avino KM, et al, editors. In: Holistic nursing: a handbook for practice. Burlington, MA: Jones & Bartlett Learning; 2020. p. 263–76.

18. Hod K, Melamed S, Dekel R, et al. Burnout, but not job strain, is associated with irritable bowel syndrome in working adults. J Psychosom Res 2020;134:110–21.

19. Melamed S, Shirom A, Toker S, et al. Burnout and risk of cardiovascular disease: evidence, possible causal paths, and promising research directions. Psychol Bull 2006;132(3):327–53.

20. Irwin MR. Sleep and inflammation: partners in sickness and in health. Nat Rev Immunol 2019;19(11):702–15.

21. Dolsen MR, Prather AA, Lamers F, et al. Suicidal ideation and suicide attempts: associations with sleep duration, insomnia, and inflammation. Psychol Med 2020;1–10.

22. Stewart NH, Arora VM. The impact of sleep and circadian disorders on physician burnout. Chest 2019;156(5):1022–30.

23. Rusch HL. Links Between Stress, Sleep, and Inflammation: A Translational Perspective of Resilience. Dissertation. Karolinska Institutet. 2020. Available at: https://www.proquest.com/docview/2497240385?pq-origsite=gscholar&fromopenview=true.

24. Leiter MP, Hakanen JJ, Ahola K, et al. Organizational predictors and health consequences of changes in burnout: A 12-year cohort study. J Organ Behav 2013; 34(7):959–73.

25. Barello S, Palamenghi L, Graffigna G. Burnout and somatic symptoms among frontline healthcare professionals at the peak of the Italian COVID-19 pandemic. Psychiatry Res 2020;290:113–29.

26. West CP, Dyrbye LN, Shanafelt TD. Physician burnout: contributors, consequences and solutions. J Intern Med 2018;283(6):516–29.

27. Zangaro G, Dulko D, Sullivan D, et al. Systematic review of burnout in U.S Nurses 2022: In print.

28. Cohen S, Kamarck T, Mermelstein R. Perceived stress scale. Measuring Stress A Guide Health Soc scientists 1994;10(2):1–2.

29. Fernández-Sánchez JC, Pérez-Mármol JM, Blásquez A, et al. Association between burnout and cortisol secretion, perceived stress, and psychopathology in palliative care unit health professionals. Palliat Support Care 2018;16(3): 286–97.

30. Derogatis LR, Lipman RS, Covi L. SCL-90. Administration, scoring and procedures manual-I for the R (revised) version and other instruments of the Psychopathology Rating Scales Series. Chicago: Johns Hopkins University School of Medicine; 1977.

31. Qiao Z, Chen L, Chen M, et al. Prevalence and factors associated with occupational burnout among HIV/AIDS healthcare workers in China: a cross-sectional study. BMC Public Health 2016;16:335.

32. Bride BE, Robinson MM, Yegidis B, et al. Development and validation of the secondary traumatic stress scale. Res Social work Pract 2004;14(1):27–35.

33. Favros C, Chene LJ, Soelch CM, et al. Mental Health Symptoms and Work-Related Stressors in Hospital Midwives and NICU Nurses: A Mixed Methods Study. Front Psychiatry 2018;9(364):1–12.

34. Zigmond AS Snaith RP. The Hospital Anxiety and Depression Scale. Acta Psychiatr Scand 1983;67:361–70.

35. Mealer M, Jones J, Newman J, et al. The presence of resilience is associated with a healthier psychological profile in intensive care unit (ICU) nurses: results of a national survey. Int J Nurs Stud 2012;49(3):292–9.

36. Connor KM, Davidson JR. Development of a new resilience scale: The Connor-Davidson resilience scale (CD-RISC). Depress Anxiety 2003;18(2):76–82.

37. Arrogante O, Aparicio-Zaldivar E. Burnout and health among critical care professionals: The mediational role of resilience. Intensive Crit Care Nurs 2017;42: 110–5.

38. Ware JE Jr, Kosinski M, Keller SD. A 12-Item Short-Form Health Survey: construction of scales and preliminary tests of reliability and validity. Med Care 1996;1: 220–33.

39. Sterling M. General health questionnaire–28 (GHQ-28). J Phys 2011;57(4):259.

40. Khamisa N, Peltzer K, Ilic D, et al. Work related stress, burnout, job satisfaction and general health of nurses: A follow-up study. Int J Nurs Pract 2016;22:538–45.

41. Fountoulakis KN, Iacovides A, Kleanthous S, et al. The greek translation of the symptoms rating scale for depression and anxiety: preliminary results of the validation study. BMC Psychiatry 2003;3(21):1–8.

42. Papathanasiou IV. Work-related mental consequences: implications of burnout on mental health status among health care providers. Acta Inform Med 2015; 23(1):22.

43. Andrich D, Schoubroeck L. The general health questionnaire: A psychometric analysis using latent trait theory. Psychol Med 1989;19(2):469–85.

44. Sacadura-Liete E, Sousa-Uva A, Rebelo-de-Andrade H, et al. Association between chronic stress and immune response to influenza vaccine in healthcare workers. Rev Port Saúde Pública 2014;32(1):18–26.
45. Ware JE Jr. SF-36 health survey. In: Maruish ME, editor. The use of psychological testing for treatment planning and outcomes assessment. Lawrence Erlbaum Associates Publishers; 1999. p. 1227–46.
46. Suner-Soler R, Grau-Martin A, Font-Mayolas S, et al. Burnout and quality of life among spanish healthcare personnel. J Psychiatr Ment Health Nurs 2013;20: 305–13.
47. Anagnostopoulos F, Niakas D. Job burnout, health-related quality of life, and sickness absence in Greek health professionals. Eur Psychol 2010;15(2):132–41.
48. McCarthy S. Post-traumatic stress diagnostic scale (PDS). Occup Med 2008; 58(5):379.
49. Marteau TM, Bekker H. The development of a six-item short-form of the state scale of the Spielberger State—Trait Anxiety Inventory (STAI). Br J Clin Psychol 1992;31(3):301–6.
50. Albini E, Zoni S, Parrinello G, et al. An integrated model for the assessment of stress-related risk factors in health care professionals. Ind Health 2011;49(1): 15–23.
51. Williams S, Cooper CL. Measuring occupational stress: development of the pressure management indicator. J Occup Health Psychol 1998;3(4):306–21.
52. Harwood L, Ridley J, Wilson B, et al. Occupational burnout, retention and health outcomes in nephrology nurses. CANNT J 2010;20(4):18–23.
53. Skorobogatova N, Žemaitienė N, Šmigelskas K, et al. Professional burnout and concurrent health complaints in neonatal nursing. Open Med (Wars) 2017;12: 328–34.
54. Alexandrova-Karamanova A, Todorova I, Montgomery A, et al. Burnout and health behaviors in health professionals from seven european countries. Int Arch Occup Environ Health 2016;89:1059–75.
55. Restauri N, Sheridan AD. Burnout and post-traumatic stress disorder in the coronavirus disease 2019 (COVID-19) pandemic: intersection, impact, and interventions. Am Coll Radiol 2020;17(7):921–6.
56. Rangachari PL, Woods J. Preserving organizational resilience, patient safety, and staff retention during COVID-19 requires a holistic consideration of the psychological safety of healthcare workers. Int J Environ Res Public Health 2020; 17(12):4267.
57. Wei H, Roberts P, Strickler J, et al. Nurse leaders' strategies to foster nurse resilience. J Nurs Manag 2019;27(4):681–7.
58. Virkstis K, Herleth A, Langr M. Cracks in the foundation of the care environment undermine nurse resilience. J Nurs Admin 2018;48(12):597–9.

Moving?

Make sure your subscription moves with you!

To notify us of your new address, find your **Clinics Account Number** (located on your mailing label above your name), and contact customer service at:

Email: journalscustomerservice-usa@elsevier.com

800-654-2452 (subscribers in the U.S. & Canada)
314-447-8871 (subscribers outside of the U.S. & Canada)

Fax number: 314-447-8029

**Elsevier Health Sciences Division
Subscription Customer Service
3251 Riverport Lane
Maryland Heights, MO 63043**

*To ensure uninterrupted delivery of your subscription, please notify us at least 4 weeks in advance of move.

Printed and bound by CPI Group (UK) Ltd, Croydon, CR0 4YY

03/10/2024

01040474-0017